THE
SINUS
CURE

By Debra Fulghum Bruce

The Snoring Cure (with Laurence A. Smolley, M.D.)

Super Calcium Counter:
The Essential Guide to Building Strong Bones
(with Harris H. McIlwain, M.D.)

Eat to Stay Young: The Anti-Aging Program
(with Catherine Christie, Ph.D., R.D., and
Susan Mitchelle, Ph.D., R.D.)

The Osteoporosis Cure:
Reverse Crippling Effects with New Treatments
(with Harris H. McIlwain, M.D.)

Breathe Right Now (with Laurence A. Smolley, M.D.)

The Fibromyalgia Handbook (with Harris H. McIlwain, M.D.)

Making a Baby: Everything You Need to Know to Get Pregnant
(with Samuel Thatcher, M.D., Ph.D.)

The Sinus Cure: Seven Simple Steps to Relieve Sinusitis
and Other Ear, Nose, and Throat Conditions
(with Murray Grossan, M.D.)

Miracle Touch

Diet for a Pain Free Life (with Harris H. McIlwain, M.D.)

Pain Free Back (with Harris H. McIlwain, M.D.)

Pain Free Arthritis (with Harris H. McIlwain, M.D.)

Reversing Osteopenia (with Harris H. McIlwain, M.D.)

THE SINUS CURE

Seven Simple Steps to Relieve Sinusitis and Other Ear, Nose, and Throat Conditions

DEBRA FULGHUM BRUCE, Ph.D.,

& MURRAY GROSSAN, M.D.

BALLANTINE BOOKS · NEW YORK

2007 Ballantine Books Trade Paperback Edition

Copyright © 2001, 2007 by Debra Fulghum Bruce, Ph.D.,
and Murray Grossan, M.D.

Published in the United States by Ballantine Books,
an imprint of The Random House Publishing Group,
a division of Random House, Inc., New York.

BALLANTINE and colophon are registered trademarks
of Random House, Inc.

Originally published in paperback in different form in the United
States by Ballantine Books, an imprint of The Random House Publishing
Group, a division of Random House, Inc., in 2001.

ISBN 978-0-345-49602-7

Printed in the United States of America

www.ballantinebooks.com

4 6 8 9 7 5 3

Text design by Holly Johnson

To our faithful support team:

Robert G. Bruce Jr., M.Div.

Rosalyn Grossan

ACKNOWLEDGMENTS

In our quest to give accurate and up-to-date information on sinus disease, we have received generous assistance, along with a wealth of breakthrough information, from a very gifted and select group of health care and support professionals. We express our gratitude to the following:

Harris H. McIlwain, M.D., with Tampa Medical Group, P.A., and Kimberly McIlwain, M.D., for insight on medical complications with sinus disease.

Lori Steinmeyer, M.S., R.D./L.D., Tampa, Florida, for nutritional consultation.

Brittnye Bruce, M.S., for up-to-date information on stress management.

Michael F. McIlwain, D.M.D., for information on dental problems with sinusitis.

Ashley Elizabeth Bruce for assistance with copywriting and proofreading skills.

Nick Ingkatanuwat for sharing his graphic art talents.

Rob Bruce III, for computer assistance and promotional consideration.

Dr. Wellington Tichenor, a New York–based allergist, whose Web site, www.sinuses.com, has provided excellent help and information.

Our agent, Denise Marcil, for believing in the need for a book on sinusitis and helping to establish our relationship with Ballantine.

A special thanks to our editors at Ballantine, Elizabeth Zack and Jillian Quint, for believing in this project and turning it into a finely edited book.

FOREWORD

You would think that with all our medical advances in the past fifty years, sinus disease would be where smallpox and malaria are today. Yet sinusitis is worse today than before the antibiotic age. Here we are starting a new century with millions of people in the United States requiring treatment for sinus conditions. These men, women, and children not only have primary sinusitis but suffer from secondary complications of asthma and pulmonary disease as a result. What has gone wrong? Why can't we prevent sinusitis?

If you go online or to your favorite mall bookstore, you will find many books on sinus disease. One current book even extols the benefits of sinus surgery. What's unique about *The Sinus Cure* is that it motivates you to get well so you can avoid surgery and the risk of complications.

Another book on sinus healing claims that if you take various combinations of different vitamins and herbs, you will be cured. While we include a section on herbs for sinus relief in this book, it is difficult to prove that herbs are cure-all drugs (in fact, sometimes herbs act like drugs on the body and can even have a harmful or toxic effect).

What about those Internet sites that appear to have all the answers to prevent and treat your sinusitis? Some are extremely well done, but mostly they deal with anatomical details and recommend seeing the doctor when you are sick. They take the need for self-care out of *your* hands and put your health in your doctor's hands! Others claim that taking this rare root from Bali or some homeopathic remedy will cure you. But you have to be sure to type in your credit card number before they'll tell you the actual name!

In this book, we present cutting-edge information on how to cure sinusitis. Health journalist and author Debra Fulghum Bruce, Ph.D., and I are of the same mind when it comes to sinusitis. We are convinced that with the right information most people can actually cure their own sinus problems.

Debra speaks from personal experience. She suffered with chronic sinusitis for years and searched everywhere for the safest remedies to clear up sinus symptoms. Debra is passionate about *The Sinus Cure* and presents the most helpful modalities in this book. In fact, since she's been using these "cures," her sinus symptoms rarely flare up.

I speak as a sinus expert. I've been a board-certified ear, nose, and throat specialist for more than forty years and have successfully treated thousands of people with all degrees of sinusitis, using the methods described in this book.

Why is my approach to treating this common problem different—and hopefully better? Let me give you some history. In 1970 I became an advanced scuba diver. I then received a certificate as a diving physician. Since that time I have specialized in' treating scuba divers' ear, nose, and throat problems. In deep diving all of your body's systems change, and the doctor has to rethink all treatments. For example, divers can't take most drugs when they dive, as drugs work differently a hundred feet under the ocean. Some professional divers are paid three hundred dollars an hour, so taking sick days off from work until the sinuses clear up is not an option. Likewise, many of the popular sinus surgeries would mean no more diving, so surgery isn't an option either. Being a diver myself, I was not going to tell a diver who suffered with sinusitis to stop diving!

In a sense, my attitude proved advantageous: I had to rethink the reason why divers couldn't clear their ears, got lightheaded, got nosebleeds, and experienced other difficulties. Out of this came several drug-free approaches to sinusitis and blocked ears. For example, I was seeing athletic divers who couldn't clear their ears. Yet on every exam they showed no disease; they had normal sinus X-rays. When I measured the movement of the cilia (tiny hairs that carry anything on their surface out of the respiratory tract), it was poor. Interestingly, when the cilia were restored, then the divers could clear their sinuses and ears easily and return to diving. From this I developed the Hydro Pulse™ Nasal/Sinus Irrigator (see page 120) as well as the use of oral enzymes that thin the mucus and clear sinus pain.

They say that necessity is the mother of invention. At my practice typically our newest patients have already had the latest antibiotics, yet they are still sick and depend on us for relief. This has forced us to develop some innovative approaches to curing sinusitis that are detailed in this book.

One of these is a technique that helps you relax and reduce stress, thus helping to reduce sinusitis. For centuries there have been places of healing—hot springs, mountain retreats, religious shrines—and in the book we explain why they work and how you can benefit in a similar manner. Another technique involves using natural fruit enzymes to help reduce inflammation and thin mucus, making it easier to drain your congested sinuses.

There are news groups on the Internet devoted to sinus patients. One of the most frequent questions these groups receive is which antibiotic to take for a sinus infection. Yet an antibiotic may fail because it is not specific for the infectious organism or the bacteria have developed resistance. However, mostly they fail because they are not undertaken in conjunction with other procedures such as drinking hot tea, resting, relaxing, and ensuring proper drainage. We will tell you how to help the antibiotic work fast and efficiently to end infection.

Furthermore, many articles appear in medical journals and in the popular press advising against the overuse of antibiotics. No one disputes that this is a true risk, but what exactly can the patient do to get well? We talk about this in the book.

You know, many people are afraid or ashamed to go to the doctor for a runny nose. They just accept and suffer with postnasal drip. But did you know that a chronic runny nose (sinusitis) can lead to chest disease and kidney or arthritic changes? Treatment—often *simple* treatment—can prevent more serious problems from occurring. In fact, many cases of sleep apnea and snoring clear up when the nose is cleared.

For forty years I have successfully taught my patients how to prevent and treat sinusitis. In this book I hope to teach a much wider audience. And as new developments take place, you can go to my Web site, www.ent-consult.com, to check on them. We want to get you well!

Last, I need to confess a bias: I am unable to recommend to my patients any therapy that hasn't been proved according to the scientific method. The scientific method means that anyone can try this medicine or device and get the same results. It means that the method is open and known and can be tried over and over again by careful observers. Thus, there are more than thirty articles that support using methods we discuss in this book, such as the Hydro Pulse Nasal/Sinus Irrigator or oral enzymes; there are even medical journal articles to support treatments like hot tea and chicken soup! Not only are the remedies provided in this book backed by medical journal studies and articles, but my own experience with many patients will qualify for a recommendation in this book. If you don't see your favorite herb here, it's not because we think that it doesn't work. Rather, it's because, according to my criteria, we are not satisfied that we can *prove* that it works.

We now give you the latest "cures" for sinusitis—treatments that really work. Be well!

—Dr. Murray Grossan
Medical Editor

CONTENTS

CONTENTS

INTRODUCTION:
ONLY YOUR NOSE KNOWS

People know I'm coming into a room by my chronic throat clearing. I've tried most prescribed medications and while I get relief for a few days, there is still a constant drip in my throat that causes me to cough or clear it. I've seen four different specialists over the past nine years. I've had two sinus surgeries, and neither did any good. In fact, I feel miserable much of the time, whether from a sore throat, nasal congestion, or postnasal drip. The days I'm not congested, I invariably have a sinus headache. Can't anyone help me?

—MEREDITH, *age forty-seven*

I live in southern California, where the temperature is hot, the air is humid, and trees bloom year round. My sinuses stay inflamed all the time. When I take decongestants, my heart races, and I feel so jittery. The medications really don't make my sinusitis any better, as I have headaches almost daily. When the pollen is high or if there is a weather change, my head and ears throb from the pressure of fluid.

*I tell my doctor that if I didn't have chronic sinusitis, I'd be
the healthiest person ever. Still, my family thinks my sinus
problems are all in my head. I tell them they are right—
literally.*

—PAUL, *age thirty-two*

It's not unusual for those around you to think your sinus symptoms are in your head. After all, chances are that you look perfectly healthy and function quite normally at home or at work.
Outwardly, no one around you can see the misery you feel. But
you know different. You know how sinus misery—the ongoing
pain, swelling, congestion, and postnasal drip—keeps you from
fully enjoying life.

No one needs to tell you of the struggles you face from lack
of restful sleep at night and the resulting inability to concentrate
during the day. You also know how the medicines taken to control these symptoms leave you nervous, fatigued, spaced out, or
just downright crabby. Chronic sinusitis can even disrupt your
career, keeping you from making a living to support yourself and
your family.

Thirty-seven-year-old Beth from Miami, Florida, had suffered chronic postnasal drip since childhood. This young trial
attorney also suffered from allergies and chronic rhinosinusitis,
long-term inflammation or swelling of the tissue lining the sinuses. Normally, sinuses are filled with air. However, when sinuses
become blocked and filled with fluid, bacteria can grow and
cause an infection.

Whenever Beth's sinuses became inflamed from environmental triggers such as pollen, mold, or chemical fumes, or if she
got a cold virus, she lived with weeks of nasal obstruction, purulent nasal drainage, and facial pain and pressure. Beth said the

perpetual postnasal drip made her cough constantly, and she even lost her voice right before two important jury trials.

Using the seven-step program outlined in this book, Beth was able to gain control of her sinusitis and reclaim her life again. Not only did she learn how to keep her nasal passages clear, she realized that she had to make some changes in her lifestyle and talk to her doctor about different medications, including a nasal steroid spray. Today, Beth has gone three years without a sinus infection, and her voice is clear and strong.

Over the past five years since we first wrote *The Sinus Cure*, there have been some revolutionary changes in the understanding and treatment of sinusitis. For example, most doctors used to treat sinusitis with antibiotics. Now we know that antibiotics are often unnecessary and if misused or overused can lead to drug-resistant supergerms that are difficult if not impossible to eradicate. We also have cutting-edge scientific substantiation on more natural therapies that help to decrease inflammation in the body and boost immune function both important for healthy sinuses. In addition, there have been groundbreaking discoveries in medical treatment and outpatient surgical procedures that were not even considered five years ago.

This revised edition of *The Sinus Cure* arms you with the accurate, up-to-date information you need to lead a healthy, active life. We hope that you and your loved ones will benefit greatly from this update.

SINUSITIS AND INFLAMMATION

Sinusitis is defined as an inflammatory process (whether infectious and/or noninfectious in origin) of the paranasal sinuses, four pairs of air-filled spaces within the bones of the skull and face. These facial cavities are located above the eyes (frontal), behind the nose in the center of the skull base (sphenoid), on either side of the face (ethmoid), and beneath the eyes in the cheek area (maxillary). The sinus cavities produce mucus, which drains through the ostia (small openings) in your nose. If the sinus cavities get clogged with mucus and the openings are blocked, infection can result.

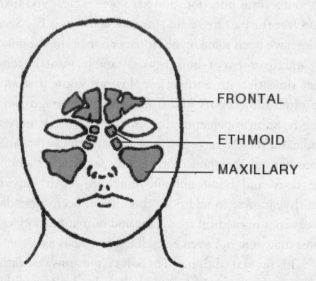

FRONTAL

ETHMOID

MAXILLARY

The Sinuses

1. *The frontal sinuses lie above your nose and just above your eyes, behind your forehead.*
2. *The maxillary sinuses are cavities located inside each cheekbone. They are the largest of the sinuses.*
3. *The ethmoids are filled with tiny air pockets and are between your eyes.*
4. *The sphenoids lie deep in your skull, behind the ethmoids.*

When conditions are healthy, it means that the mucus in your sinuses is pushed out of the nose by cilia, tiny hairs that beat or wave rhythmically to carry anything on their surface in the direction of their motion out of the respiratory tract. This mucus provides a highway for the good white cells produced by your body to reach any invading bad bacteria. It also cleans the air you breathe, moistens your sinuses, and then slides down the back of your throat to your stomach, where acid destroys the mucus and trapped bacteria.

When conditions are not healthy, you get sinusitis. This happens when your cilia slow down or stop working properly. Or sinusitis can occur when there is an anatomical blockage and the stagnant mucus becomes infected.

HOW PREVALENT IS SINUSITIS?

Chronic sinusitis—that is, sinusitis that continues for weeks or months—is the most prevalent adult disease in the United States and is estimated to affect more than 38 million Americans. With an increase in population along with the increase in pollution and drug-resistant bacteria, the number of people who suffer from chronic sinus problems continues to skyrocket.

SIGNS AND SYMPTOMS OF SINUSITIS

Coughing all night because of the continuous, thick postnasal drip running down the back of your throat; a throbbing earache because of trapped fluid; the excruciating pain of pounding headaches; chronic hoarseness from clearing your throat repeatedly—the discomfort of sinusitis is all too familiar to millions.

Besides the headache pain and pressure, postnasal drip, and congestion, there are other problems associated with sinus disease. You may feel achy and fatigued and suffer from ear pain or sore throat. Many individuals have fever with a sinus infection. Or your teeth may hurt, making you think you have dental problems. As an example, thirty-seven-year-old Raymond went to two different dentists seeking relief for throbbing upper molars. "About three of my molars started hurting after I got over a horrible head cold," he said. "At first it was a dull ache, but after a few days my whole jaw was throbbing, my head was pounding, and I had a fever."

After agreeing that his teeth were perfectly healthy, the second dentist referred Raymond to an ear, nose, and throat doctor (ENT). The ENT diagnosed him with a bacterial sinus infection and started him on antibiotics and a decongestant.

Fortunately for Raymond, the dentist referred him to a specialist for an accurate diagnosis and treatment. Within a week, his pain had subsided and he felt more like himself. Sadly, in some situations people go for months thinking they have a bad tooth, or tension or migraine headaches, when in fact they are suffering from the signs of chronic sinusitis. As a side note, an infected upper tooth can sometimes lead to a serious sinus infection that is difficult to resolve.

A STRONG SINUSITIS/ASTHMA LINK

Not only can your sinuses affect tissue in your teeth, face, and jaw, causing excruciating pain, but sinusitis can also trigger an all-out asthma attack. Did you know that more than 50 percent of all asthmatics also suffer from chronic sinusitis at some point, which can make asthma symptoms flare up and worsen?

Chronic sinusitis can sometimes damage the nasal membrane or structure, requiring corrective surgery to regain function. Left untreated, sinusitis may lead to meningitis, an infection of the brain that can lead to brain damage. In some rare cases, a blood clot forms in veins around the sinuses (cavernous sinus thrombosis) and can affect the brain like a stroke.

If you have any signs or symptoms of sinusitis, talk with your doctor to be sure no other problems are present. Sinus disease is serious and should certainly not be taken lightly.

COST IN PAIN AND SUFFERING

While chronic sinusitis causes tremendous physical suffering, it is also an expensive illness, resulting in more than 16 million visits to doctors' offices annually for treatment. In fact, during the three-year period from 1989 to 1992, annual expenditures on prescription medications for sinusitis rose from $50 million to $200 million. Remember Raymond? He had not met his insurance deductible, so his diagnosis of sinusitis cost more than $500 out of pocket to pay for the dental consultations, the ENT visit, and the medications. Add to this unexpected cost the income he lost from missing work. Combined with expensive treatments, the cost of personal suffering is great not only for patients but also for their families, friends, employers, and co-workers.

THE COST OF ADDED STRESS

The stress of sinusitis not only is associated with feeling miserable but extends to doctors' visits, medical bills, cost of medications, and missed days at work or school. Another great cause of stress is the anxiety and worry about whether you will ever feel better. Over a period of time, these stressors can result in depression and other emotional reactions that further limit your ability to deal effectively with life. Many sinus sufferers cannot exercise outdoors because of pollen or dust allergies. Some sinus sufferers cannot enjoy a day at the beach because of high humidity, or a mountain hike because of cold, damp air. Still others are just too fatigued to move around much because they ache all over from low-grade infection, or the medication they take zaps any energy or motivation for exercise. This inability to enjoy life and exercise can lead to feelings of malaise or depression that only add to your lethargic state.

THE HIGH COST OF PERSONAL SUFFERING

What do you feel when you notice your sinuses becoming inflamed or irritated? Other than the common symptoms of headache, pressure, swelling, congestion, and postnasal drip, there are more serious personal repercussions experienced by millions of sinus sufferers every day of their life. Do any of these statements describe you?

- I dread getting up each day knowing that I have to live with this chronic and annoying problem.
- I don't want to talk to anyone—even my family members—when I have sinus headaches.
- When my sinuses flare up, I get muscle aches and pains throughout my body. I end up canceling any social activities and even miss a few days of work because I feel so miserable.
- My sinus problems affect my work performance and my relationship with colleagues.
- I feel overall fatigue that does not go away even after several large cups of strongly caffeinated coffee.
- I feel in a low mood that does not lift even as I get on with my daily activities.
- I have felt depressed enough to ask my doctor for antidepressants.
- I feel irritable and impatient, and I have mood swings from the sinus medications.
- I often have difficulty being with a large group, as I feel jittery and nervous from the medications I take.
- The medications I take make it difficult for me to concentrate in school or at work.
- I am unable to recall useful information after being up all night with a sinus headache, and I sometimes feel "foggy."

IT'S TIME TO FIND ANSWERS

So you've felt the fatigue, fogginess, and irritability sinus disease can cause. Maybe you have lived with a plugged-up nose and annoying postnasal drip for years. You've read the self-help books, and your doctor has prescribed the latest medications. You've even gone online searching for breakthrough treatments. Yet you still suffer and are looking for answers, a possible cure.

Before we share answers in this book, let's address what a "sinus cure" means. A cure is defined as partial or complete relief of symptoms. Therefore, after years of research, interviews, and personal and professional experience, we wrote this book to share cures from the top health care specialists, and patients—cures that really work. Although medical research has yet to find a definitive cure to end sinusitis, the treatments and medications described in this book will work in most cases to greatly reduce or end your sinus problems. The conventional and alternative modalities we discuss are effective, and most of them have no side effects.

Most important to understand is that there is no one-size-fits-all approach when it comes to managing your sinusitis. Finding the remedies that work best in your situation may take some time—and trial and error. But once you find what works to minimize your symptoms and keep infections at bay, your quality of life will soar—and that we promise!

HOW THIS BOOK CAN HELP

Unlike other books on the subject of sinusitis, *The Sinus Cure* places you, the reader, at center stage by focusing on your personal risk factors for sinusitis. As you read, you will see that we quickly move beyond a description of sinusitis and related disorders such as asthma, allergy, and gastroesophageal reflux disease (GERD) to personalized self-help solutions that you can use right now to reduce your problem with sinusitis and, ultimately, minimize your symptoms altogether without dependency on prescribed medications or antibiotics.

Here's how we'll accomplish this. In chapter 1, "What Is Sinusitis?" we explain the anatomical parts of the body that are necessary for healthy breathing and how sinusitis can develop when any of these parts malfunction. In this key chapter, we discuss how sinusitis is linked with other problems such as postnasal drip, sinobronchial syndrome, and asthma and how getting in control of the sinusitis symptoms and/or infection can help to reduce the other problems.

We will address the various ailments related to sinusitis in chapter 2, "Sinusitis and Coexisting Problems." We'll also discuss some doctor's recommendations you might consider to reduce the occurrence of these coexisting problems so you can enjoy a greater quality of life.

Chapter 3, "Sinus Pain . . . and What You Can Do to End It," explains some painful conditions such as sinus headache, earache, and sore throat that you might experience along with sinusitis. We'll give you the signs and symptoms, as well as some easy methods of treating these common painful disorders to help you get on the mend fast!

We start our program immediately in "Step 1: Make the Diagnosis," and take you on a virtual appointment with an ENT (ear, nose, and throat doctor). We will explain the physical examination and how the doctor will proceed to make a diagnosis, using a scope with a special lens to check your sinuses, evaluating the glands in your neck, assessing the temporomandibular joint (TMJ), and peering into your ears and throat to see if there might be associated problems causing the congestion and/or headache. Different screening tests such as computed tomography (CT) scans are used to make a correct diagnosis, and we'll explain these tests and what they might indicate.

"Step 2: Try Nasal Irrigation" is a must-read for every sinus sufferer. In this key step we explain how a simple method of cleaning your sinuses daily with saline solution helps to remove bacteria-ridden mucus and can help you avoid sinus infections altogether. Nasal irrigation also helps to heal sluggish cilia, which are vital to keep mucus flowing naturally.

In "Step 3: Consider Complementary Treatments," we'll go into detail about effective alternative therapies, such as hydrotherapy, herbal therapies, homeopathy, acupressure, massage, and even the power of belief, that can be used to boost sinus health and your immunity. For instance, one alternative method is taking papaya enzyme tablets bucally (holding them inside the mouth between the inside of your cheek and the gum) four times daily to reduce inflammation and liquefy mucus (see page 207). Some alternative treatments, such as natural dietary supplements or botanicals can be purchased over the counter at your supermarket or health food store, while others, including chiropractic and acupuncture, may require the work of a trained professional. But all these therapies have helped sinusitis sufferers and may help you, too.

"Step 4: Clean Up the Air around You" will teach you some practical ways to take control of your home and work environment to reduce sinus symptoms. This step will help you identify and understand some of the triggers that set you up for sinus congestion, sore throat, wheezing or coughing, headache, and a constant runny nose, among other symptoms. These triggers may be allergens (pollens, mold, pet dander, dust mites), irritants (smoke, chemical sprays, odors), and/or physical changes (cold air, weather fronts, exercise). No matter what triggers your sinus symptoms, managing the trigger is vital to controlling and even halting sinus problems.

We will explain the role proper nourishment plays in avoiding chronic sinusitis in "Step 5: Boost Healing Nutrients." In this step, we discuss how to eat for optimal sinus health and give you the latest studies on specific nutrients necessary to boost immune function and increase healing. Some of these nutrients, such as antioxidants, flavonoids, and omega-3 fatty acids, are known to decrease inflammation and may allow you to take fewer medications. We'll also give some simple dietary strategies that can help improve symptoms. For instance, one strategy is to sip hot tea to help thin mucus and keep the cilia moving naturally. Another helpful strategy is to avoid all iced drinks, which can damage cilia, causing them to stop functioning altogether (see pages 7–9).

Prepare for downtime in "Step 6: De-Stress to Stay Well," as we elaborate on some easy mind/body therapies and how they can help you keep your life—and daily stress—in perspective and even improve immune function so the chance of infection decreases. Because chronic stress tears down the immune system, increasing the chance of a sinus infection, this step will let you become your own bodyguard by learning relaxation techniques and strategies for sounder sleep to help your body stay well.

"Step 7: Use Effective Medical Therapies" will educate you on the latest medications that are used to treat—even cure—the symptoms of sinusitis and related problems. We will give you current information on using nasal inhalers, nasal sprays, and oral medications, explaining why the medication will help and how to take it properly to halt or even reverse your sinus symptoms. Along with a discussion on the latest medications for sinus symptoms, we'll explain how we all must be extremely vigilant about taking antibiotics properly and avoid overusing these medications.

In chapter 11, "What If Your Doctor Says . . . Surgery?" we will give you the latest information on various types of nasal and sinus surgery, including the new balloon sinoplasty. We want you to review the pros and cons of surgery so that you can work with your doctor and make the best decision for your situation.

Read on and continue to learn how to manage your sinus problem in an orderly manner. Talk with your doctor for specific advice on your own situation, and join thousands of people who have learned to manage their sinus problems and are enjoying life again.

HOW THIS BOOK CAN TRULY HELP YOU

In *The Sinus Cure*, sinus sufferers from around the world have shared the best natural treatments, which are described in Steps 1–6. These methods, along with effective breakthrough medicines discussed in Step 7, can offer dramatic improvement in your sinus symptoms and quality of life without the side effects of drowsiness, stomach upset, or nervousness caused by the older sinus drugs.

We encourage you to talk with your doctor and seek an accurate medical diagnosis. Once you understand the causes of your particular sinus problem and know which treatments are most likely to be effective, you can begin to manage sinusitis just as you do other areas of your life.

While you are checking on natural therapies for sinusitis, ask your doctor about nasal steroid inhalers that reduce inflammation, as well as other safe and effective medications to reduce congestion. Using the inhaled medicine, along with healing foods, natural supplements, increased exercise, and sounder sleep, can help you to heal your sinuses, boost your immune function, and keep infection at bay.

YOUR SINUS CURE GOAL

Sinusitis is an extremely common problem that many doctors believe is incurable. Fortunately, in this book we highlight conventional and complementary remedies that may prove them wrong! Your goal should be to get in control of all sinus symptoms—inflammation, headache, pressure, swelling, congestion, and postnasal drip—so you can do the activities you wish without thinking about your sinusitis symptoms. Whether your sinus problems are mild, moderate, or severe, acute or chronic, you can regain control if you follow the advice in this book.

Who has time for sinus pain or pressure, much less the ongoing symptoms of cough and congestion? Certainly not you! To that end, this book will provide you with groundbreaking information and the most effective natural therapies and effective medications you need to make sinusitis a problem of your past.

Let's get started!

Part One

ALL ABOUT SINUSITIS

Chapter 1

WHAT IS SINUSITIS?

I never think about breathing . . . until my sinuses act up. Then when I can't breathe through my nose, have difficulty swallowing, and the constant drainage of thick mucus makes me gag, breathing is the only thing I think about! How could something that makes my life so miserable be so important?

—JUSTINE, *age thirty-nine*

Millions of sinus sufferers share Justine's frank appraisal of her upper airway problems. Even though sinus symptoms are disturbing and steal quality of life, your upper respiratory system is a very complicated and vital structure. Not only is it responsible for your voice production, swallowing, and keeping the back of the throat clear of food and mucus, it helps to prepare the air you breathe to go into your lungs—to keep your body functioning as a fine-tuned machine.

In this chapter, we will introduce you to some breathing basics to help you understand what is happening anatomically when you breathe clearly—and when you don't. We'll explain how the sinuses function correctly and some key factors that cause them to function poorly, such as a viral infection, dry heat, or a refreshing glass of iced tea in the summertime (iced drinks slow the nasal cilia that are crucial to keep mucus flowing; see pages 7–9). After we discuss various types of sinusitis—acute, chronic, and fungal—we'll reveal risk factors that can increase your chance of having sinus problems. Finally, we'll explain the connection between the increasingly common gastroesophageal reflux disease (GERD) and sinusitis and give you some sage advice on how to stop this problem from robbing you of your sleep, your voice, and your ability to breathe clearly and be active.

BREATHING BASICS

Within your upper airway there are about twenty muscles that are responsible for carrying out daily functions, as well as for maintaining the opening of the airway, even when external factors tend to make it close or collapse. Specialized muscles in the walls of the upper airway and in the surrounding tissues must keep the airway open as you breathe in and out. These muscles make sure food goes down the right way while you breathe.

Your vocal cords are a stopcock that closes so food doesn't enter your lungs. This system allows you to talk and eat at the same time. To speak, the muscles of the larynx (the voice box) tense, vibrate, open, and close the vocal cords. Fortunately, this is all done automatically without you worrying about it. (A word of caution: never laugh heartily while eating. Your system can't handle eating, breathing, and laughing all at once.)

Your Body's Thermostat

Your nose also acts as an air conditioner for your body and functions to protect your lower airway from cold or contaminated air. That's because the air you breathe varies in temperature, humidity, and purity. The nose adjusts this air temperature so that it becomes close to body temperature during its passage through the nose. Simultaneously, air humidity is modified, and particles in the air are filtered out.

How does it do this? Well, the septum divides the inside of your nose into two parts. There are also three tubular structures called turbinates that project into the nasal chambers and increase the surface areas of the walls of the inside of the nose. A mucous membrane rich in blood vessels covers these turbinates. The turbinates may swell and cause nasal obstruction, which can be caused by a variety of conditions, and usually seems worse when you are lying down. This is because the tissue fluids and blood tend to pool in your head when you recline.

The turbinates serve to warm and filter the air you breathe. They catch bacteria, viruses, toxins, and chemicals before they reach the lungs and also moisten the air. Turbinates also function to aid sleep. Normally during sleep, you turn about fifty times a night. If you didn't, you would develop pressure sores. This turning of your body also helps to distribute the body's lymph fluids.

For example, when you lie on your right side, the turbinates on the right side of your nose fill up simply by gravitational pull. When they fill to the extent that they reach the septum in the midline and apply pressure here, your body responds by turning over to the left side. Eventually the left side fills by the pull of gravity and presses on the septum, forcing you to feel uncomfortable and roll over again.

Mucus or Mucous?

It's easy to confuse the words *mucous* and *mucus*. Although they sound the same, they have distinct meanings. *Mucous* (adjective) means "covered with mucus" or "containing mucus." The *mucous membrane* is a soft, pink, skin-like structure that lines many cavities and tubes in the body, such as the respiratory tract. The mucous membrane secretes a fluid containing *mucus* (noun), a viscid, slippery secretion, which helps to lubricate and protect certain parts of the body. The mucous membranes produce between a pint and quart of mucus daily. Normal mucus contains the good stuff—lysozyme enzymes, good white cells, good allergy fighters—and is thin enough to be moved by the nasal cilia.

For those who sleep poorly, your doctor may recommend correcting a deviated septum. If the septum is badly deviated to one side, you will not experience the turbinate pressing on the septum. Instead, you will awaken feeling as if you slept on the wrong side! Just another downside to the related problems of sinusitis . . .

The Sinuses Filter Air

The sinuses are hollow cavities within your cheekbones, around and behind your nose and eyes; they are lined with mucous membranes. The four pairs of sinuses, or cavities in the head (paranasal sinuses), serve an important purpose, helping to lighten the skull and improve the tonality of your voice. They also serve as an air filter for your lungs by warming, moistening, and filtering the air in your nasal cavity. Your eyes and ears have to be positioned right where they are for binocular vision and good hearing. If the sinus cavity were solid, your head would weigh considerably more and require more muscles and bony support.

The sinuses are to blame for your never-ending production of mucus—and for people with sinus problems, this may be a lot!

Cilia Sweep Away Mucus

The entire lining of the nose is covered with a thin coat of mucus. The mucus rests on top of the cilia, tiny hairs on the cells making up the mucous membrane. The cilia beat or wave rhythmically to carry anything on their surface in the direction of their motion out of the respiratory tract. The mucus they carry is sticky and collects tiny airborne particles. This coating also contains enzymes that destroy most bacteria. Nasal cilia beat backward toward the nasopharynx. Once nasal mucus is propelled into the nasopharynx, it is swallowed for disposal into the stomach. The sinuses, Eustachian tubes, bronchi, and bronchioles also have cilia that help propel mucus.

Each of the sinuses has an ostium, a bony opening, through which the mucus drains. The cilia beat or wave in such a manner as to direct mucus and other respiratory tract secretions toward the ostium. For healthy sinuses to function optimally, this natural pattern of mucociliary clearance is essential.

Eighty-five to 90 percent of the particles inhaled nasally are blocked and removed in the nose and nasopharynx. Yet smaller particles may get into the lower respiratory tract. When the ac-

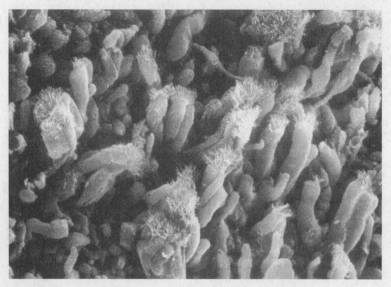

Cilia are tiny hairs that beat or wave rhythmically to carry anything on their surface in the direction of their motion out of the respiratory tract.

tion of the mucous coat is altered by trauma, drying, irritating chemicals, or any other factor, the nose, sinuses, and lower respiratory tract become more susceptible to infection.

Cilia are very sensitive to toxins and can be damaged or slowed due to

- Antihistamines
- Iced drinks
- Dryness
- Getting chilled
- Codeine
- Cocaine

> ## Healthy Cilia = Healthy Sinuses
>
> - Humidify air to the lungs
> - Trap bacteria and prevent them from entering the cells
> - Dilute bacteria and carcinogens
> - Aid the smell mechanisms
> - Help maintain proper temperature in the respiratory system
> - Provide a healthy way for good white cells to travel to attack bacteria

- Chlorine gas
- Chromium dust
- Formaldehyde

Using specialized tests, as we describe in chapter 4 (Step 1 of our program), your doctor can find out the condition of your cilia. Studies show that decreased mucociliary flow is a regular precursor to sinusitis and lower respiratory infections. In severe asthma (see page 56), the cilia of the chest are slowed as well.

HOW SINUSITIS DEVELOPS

To fight off infection and stay healthy, your sinuses must have proper mucus movement and a functioning immune system. When these are compromised, sinusitis results. Sinusitis begins when the nasal mucous membranes become "twitchy" or irritated by such triggers as

- A cold or viral infection
- Air pollution, smog
- Smoke
- Airborne allergens
- Dry or cold air
- Ozone

This irritation results in inflammation or swelling of the mucous membranes and causes your mucous glands to secrete even more mucus in an attempt to dilute the offending material. Under perfect conditions, all the mucus passes through thin ducts (about the diameter of a pencil lead) and out toward the natural ostium. A series of narrow bony openings and clefts called the osteomeatal complex (OMC) serves as the common drainage path for the frontal, maxillary, and ethmoid sinuses. However, when the OMC pathway becomes obstructed because of allergy, viral infections, nasal polyps, or pollution, it becomes inflamed.[1] This swelling causes the cilia to slow down and the sinus ostia to become obstructed, and the mucus can't drain out. The stagnant mucus then backs up into the sinuses, and because it is no longer being flushed out, it can easily become infected, affecting your nose, eyes, or middle ear, not to mention the overall body aches you may feel. With a blockage you get a vacuum effect that is painful, which is part of the sinus headache. If you've already had one or two sinus infections, you become easy prey for another.

With sinusitis, you may have thick or colored nasal drainage, facial swelling, tremendous pressure in your nose and

---

Kids and Sinusitis

Even though the sinuses are narrower in kids than in adults up until around age twelve, sinusitis is just as common in kids as in adults. Many people mistake sinusitis in kids for a cold or allergies when, in fact, the child needs specific medical attention for the sinuses. If left untreated, sinusitis can last for months, causing the child to feel generally fatigued, irritable, and inattentive in school. Sinusitis can also lead to bronchial problems and asthma.

---

eyes, head congestion, a headache, or a toothache. Sometimes all you feel is a plugged-up nose, fatigue, and flu-like aching.

TYPES OF SINUSITIS

Although some people suffer from sinusitis year round, it is most common during the winter months and may be acute, chronic, or allergic fungal.

Acute Sinusitis

Acute sinusitis usually results from a viral infection such as the common cold (called viral rhinosinusitis) or a bacterial infection. Symptoms of acute sinusitis include the following:

- Cold symptoms for more than ten days
- Nasal congestion
- Purulent nasal discharge
- Facial pain or pressure (worsens when bending over)
- Headache
- Fever
- Halitosis
- Fatigue
- Facial swelling
- Pain in upper molars
- Cough
- Ear pain and/or ear fullness

It's important to distinguish between the acute viral rhino-sinusitis of colds and secondary bacterial infections, as the treatment is vastly different. According to the Centers for Disease Control and Prevention (CDC), acute bacterial sinusitis has the following signs: maxillary pain or tenderness in the face or teeth, persistent nasal discharge, fatigue, and fever that persists beyond seven days without improvement and symptoms regardless of duration.[2] Viral infections are less severe and start to improve in seven days.

While antibiotics are effective in treating some cases of acute bacterial sinusitis, these medications are *ineffective* in viral conditions. Treatment for viral rhinosinusitis is directed at suppressing symptoms, particularly the runny nose that leads to nose blowing.

If you experience signs of a lingering cold or any of the symptoms listed above, call your doctor to see if you might have a bacterial infection. We'll provide some natural methods to reduce the chance of bacterial infections in our seven-step program, but always check with your doctor to see if medical treatment is necessary.

Chronic Sinusitis

Chronic sinusitis, the most commonly diagnosed chronic illness in the United States, feels like an ongoing cold—your nose keeps running and running. It affects more than 38 million Americans, and reports show that it is rapidly increasing in incidence.[3] Chronic sinusitis is defined as inflammation of the mucosa of the nose and paranasal sinuses lasting for at least twelve consecutive weeks.[4] These are three common symptoms of chronic sinusitis: pressure or headache, nasal obstruction or congestion, and nasal drainage or postnasal drip, particularly mucus, discolored or clear, draining down the back of the nose and the throat. This usually results in a chronic cough and/or sore throat at night. These annoying symptoms greatly interfere with restful sleep, and you may feel fatigue or malaise during daytime hours.

The goal of treating chronic sinusitis is to increase sinus drainage and resolve the offending bacteria. Daily nasal irrigation with saline solution is a superb way to keep the nasal passage clear, as you rinse out the thick mucus that builds up in the cavities. Your doctor may also recommend antibiotics to eradicate the bacteria, oral corticosteroids, topical steroids, decongestants (oral and nasal sprays), and other therapies such as mucolytic agents (expectorants), which thin mucus and promote sinus drainage. In more serious cases, surgery is used to restore sinus drainage.

Factors That May Result in Chronic Sinusitis

Allergic rhinitis
Cilia dysfunction
Cystic fibrosis
Deviated nasal septum
Dry heat
Foreign body causing obstruction (especially in
   children)
Immunodeficiency
Industrial toxins such as chromium, nickel, solvents
Microorganisms (viruses, bacteria, fungi)
Nonallergic rhinitis
Previous sinus surgery
Sick building syndrome from mold or toxins
Smoking and environmental pollutants
Trauma

Fungal Sinusitis

Fungal sinusitis encompasses a wide variety of fungal infections that range from benign, noninvasive fungal diseases that may be irritating at worst to fungal diseases that become rapidly serious.

It is thought that when a fungus is in the nose or sinuses, the body's natural defense mechanism (the eosinophils) produces too much toxin trying to kill the fungus and that this toxin (called major basic protein) is what makes the patient sick. The therapy tries to eliminate the fungus and thus stop the eosinophils' reaction. The most common fungi, those in the genera Alternaria and Cladosporium, can usually be successfully treated with antifungal medications.

It is important to realize that mold and fungi are everywhere, with more than 200,000 distinct species. Walk in the woods or enter almost any home and you will find some.

A common type of fungal sinusitis called *opportunistic fungal sinusitis* results after extensive antibiotic use. The normal bacteria are no longer there to combat the fungus, and so there is significant fungal growth. This is similar to the vaginal or oral yeast infection (thrush) that may develop after antibiotic use.

Along with opportunistic fungal sinusitis, there is allergic fungal sinusitis, fungus balls (mycetomas), and invasive fungal sinusitis, all of which require more invasive medical treatment.

Allergic fungal sinusitis (AFS) is a benign fungal disease caused by a hypersensitivity reaction to the fungi in the paranasal sinuses. Patients with allergic fungal sinusitis usually have obstruction of the sinuses caused by nasal polyps, inflamed mucosa, or a deviated septum. The obstruction causes the mucus to thicken, stagnate, and become infected. Most patients also have a history of allergy and/or asthma. In more than 75 percent of cases of AFS, the fungi implicated belong to the genera Bipolaris, Curvularia, Drechslera, Exserohilum, or Alternaria. Aspergillus species were once thought to be the major cause of allergic fungal sinusitis, but recent studies show this species accounts for only 10 to 20 percent of the cases.

The treatment of AFS involves removing any obstructions (polyps) to allow for drainage of the inflammatory material, along with oral corticosteroids for two to four weeks after the obstruction has been removed.

Fungus balls (*mycetomas*) often involve the maxillary sinus. Patients may have symptoms of chronic sinutisis with the involvement of only one sinus and may have foul-smelling breath. In addition to radiological abnormalities, thick pus or a clay-like substance is found in the sinuses. Surgery is required to remove the fungus ball, and oral corticosteroids are usually not necessary.

Invasive fungal sinusitis is found in immunocompromised patients such as those with AIDS or diabetes or who have had a bone marrow transplant. This type of fungal sinusitis progresses rapidly and typically necessitates surgery, often on an emergency basis. The fungi most often implicated in invasive sinusitis are species of Aspergillus, Fusarium, Zygomycetes (order Mucorales), and dematiaceous molds. Because this type of fungal sinusitis can invade bone, a change in vision or swelling around the eye may be the first sign.

The probability that you have any of these types of fungal sinusitis is small. On the other hand, if your sinus condition is not clearing with medications and daily nasal irrigation, then talk to your doctor. It may indicate the need for further testing and even surgery to help make the diagnosis and resolve the problem.

While the over-the-counter remedies may provide some relief, they are not effective against inflammation. Antibiotics are effective only against bacterial infections and do nothing for this chronic fungal condition. In fact, the antibiotics may contribute to producing antibiotic-resistant strains of bacteria, allowing the fungus to develop in the sinuses. Research into the treatments of fungal sinusitis is ongoing and much needed.

YOUR PREDISPOSITION TO SINUSITIS

When the openings in your sinuses become blocked or plugged up, pain and pressure start. This does not happen randomly. Rather, there are usually risk factors that predispose you to sinus problems and infection, including:

- Toxins from infections, flu, or common cold
- Allergies
- Anatomical or structural problems
- Environmental irritants
- Family history
- Immunodeficiency
- Emotional stress
- Gastroesophageal reflux disease (GERD)
- Blowing the nose too hard; sniffing too hard

Let's look at some of these common reasons for sinusitis to understand why they increase the risk of suffering with this common problem.

TOXINS FROM INFECTIONS, FLU, OR THE COMMON COLD

Everyone knows what cold misery feels like. In fact, adults can expect to get an average of three colds a year, while children may get as many as six to ten colds per year. Rhinoviruses are the most frequent causes of colds, with more than a hundred types that cause 10 to 40 percent of colds. The coronaviruses and respiratory syncytial virus (RSV) cause 20 and 10 percent, respectively.[5]

These viruses may also affect your airways, sinuses, throat, voice box, and bronchial tubes. When the aggravating symptoms of a stuffy head and nasal drainage continue for one, two, and then three weeks, the chances are great that your cold has changed to sinusitis.

What You May Feel

A cold usually begins abruptly with great discomfort in your throat followed by symptoms such as clear nasal discharge, sneezing, a tired sensation (malaise), and sometimes fever. Postnasal drip causes the sore throat and cough that accompany colds.

Colds are usually self-limiting and last around seven days. Occasionally they require antibiotics when you also have a bacterial infection. Fatigue, stress, or the virus itself may promote infection, which can weaken the body's immune system.

Distinguishing Sinusitis from a Cold or Flu

Sometimes you might mistake a cold virus for allergic rhinitis (hay fever) or a sinus infection. If your symptoms begin quickly and are over within one to two weeks, then it is usually a cold, not allergy or sinusitis. If your cold symptoms last longer than two weeks, check with your doctor to see if further testing and treatment are necessary.

With a cold, you may have thick yellow or green mucus that resolves into thin, clear mucus after a few days. A sinus infection may be different: the mucus stays thick and discolored until you begin treatment, usually antibiotic therapy. Many of the treatments explained in this book may help reduce the need for antibiotic therapy if started at the first signs of cold or infection.

To determine if what you have is a cold or the flu, take your temperature. A mild case of the flu often mimics a cold. Unlike the flu, a cold virus rarely raises your temperature above 101°F. Influenza is an acute respiratory infection caused by a variety of influenza viruses and often involves muscle aches and soreness, headache, and fever. If it is flu, you will feel some pain in your muscles. You normally do not feel muscle pain with a sinus infection. Flu viruses enter your body through the mucous membranes of the nose, eyes, or mouth. Initially the virus gets on your hand from some sick person. Every time you touch your hand to one of these areas, you are possibly infecting yourself with a virus, which makes it very important to keep your hands germ-free with frequent washing.

Seeking treatment for colds and flu in the elderly, the very young, or the chronically ill is important. If your doctor says no antibiotics are needed for a cold or flu, that is the truth. Antibiotics only work against bacterial infections. Viruses cause most colds, flu, and sore throats—and antibiotics do not work against these infections. If the cold or flu develops into a secondary infection, such as bacterial bronchitis or an ear infection, your doctor may then prescribe an antibiotic.

Newer prescription treatments such as Tamiflu and Relenza are highly effective at reducing the duration of flu symptoms if taken early in the course of the infection. Call your doctor if you have been exposed to the flu virus and suspect that your symptoms indicate the flu.

Remember, flu vaccines are recommended annually for anyone with respiratory problems, those with certain chronic illnesses, and particular high-risk groups such as health care providers and those older than age sixty-five. Ask your doctor if this may help you.

Annual Cold Statistics

While the average adult has from two to three colds and influenza-like illnesses annually, the average child has six to ten. This represents approximately 1 billion acute respiratory illnesses annually in the United States alone. Approximately 0.5 to 2 percent of colds and influenza-like illnesses are complicated by acute bacterial sinusitis in adults.[6]

ALLERGIES AND SINUSITIS

Inflammation or swelling of the nasal mucous membrane is called *rhinitis*. Allergic rhinitis is the single most common chronic allergic disease and affects more than 58 million people in the United States. A recent nationwide survey revealed that more than half (54.6 percent) of all U.S. citizens test positive to one or more allergens and 20 percent of the population suffer from daily symptoms. Allergy symptoms are the sixth-leading cause of chronic illness, with an estimated $18 billion annual health care cost.[7]

If you have allergic rhinitis, you may be predisposed to sinusitis. In fact, up to 80 percent of those with sinusitis have allergies. Unlike with colds and other respiratory infections, an overreaction of the immune system to an ordinarily harmless substance causes allergy. Substances known as allergens trigger these allergic responses.

Allergic Rhinitis (Hay Fever)

Allergic rhinitis or hay fever is triggered by antibodies that induce the body's immune cells to release histamines in response to contact with allergens. Histamines are substances in the body that cause nasal stuffiness and dripping in a cold or hay fever, bronchoconstriction in asthma, and itchy spots in a skin allergy. The most common allergens enter the body through the airway.

What You May Feel

With allergic rhinitis, you may feel a constant runny nose, ongoing sneezing, swollen nasal passages, excessive mucus, weepy eyes, and a scratchy palate and throat. A cough may result from postnasal drip. Some people with allergic rhinitis feel only a drippy nose; others are so congested that the allergy affects every part of their lives. You can often identify a child who has allergic rhinitis by the crease on the top of the nose from constant wiping (allergic salute) or dark circles under the eyes (allergic shiners).

Blocked ears and fluid in the ears because of blocked Eustachian tubes are two common results of allergic rhinitis in both adults and children. Unending fatigue is another problem and is currently receiving much attention. Some researchers believe that allergic rhinitis and chronic fatigue syndrome have a common linkage. Whether this is so or not, when you take into account nighttime congestion and medication side effects, allergic rhinitis can cause you to feel tired all the time.

What Causes Allergic Rhinitis?

Blame Mom, Dad, or the family dog for your allergies. Just as with sinusitis or even asthma, your family history (inherited genetic makeup) may also predispose you to allergies.

You are supposed to sneeze when you are exposed to very heavy dust; the sneeze gets rid of the material in your nose. But with an allergy, you sneeze with just a small amount of dust. Yet there also must be frequent exposure to allergens, such as dust mites, cockroaches, animals, pollen, or mold, to stimulate the allergic reaction. The problem arises when someone with respiratory allergies meets an allergy trigger, or allergen, and a reaction takes place.

A current theory called the *hygiene hypothesis* blames higher rates of allergies in Western countries on our high standard of cleanliness. This theory postulates that a child's immune system requires stimulation to prevent an imbalance resulting in allergies, asthma, and even autoimmune diseases such as rheumatoid arthritis and diabetes. According to the hygiene hypothesis, our immune system is like a set of scales. When the scales are balanced, we are in optimal health. But when the scale is tipped far enough, it can result in declining health or chronic or life-threatening illness. Many experts believe that the increased use of disinfectants and antibiotics may have confused our immune systems. The theory is that if you are exposed to more germs as a child—such as by having older siblings, attending day care, or being raised on a farm—then you're less likely to develop allergies or asthma. In areas where children have been given antibiotics for every sniffle or sneeze, we see a higher incidence of allergies. Children who have pets in the house in infancy may be less likely to become allergic to that type of animal. But if pets

Allergy 101

- *Mast cells* are the allergy-causing cells in the mucous lining of the nose, sinuses, and bronchi that contain chemicals such as histamine and leukotrienes.
- *Histamine* is the substance that causes nasal stuffiness and dripping in a cold or hay fever, bronchoconstriction in asthma, and itchy spots in a skin allergy.
- *Immunoglobulin E (IgE)* is the most important antibody produced during an allergic reaction. While everyone makes IgE, people who have a genetic predisposition toward an allergy make larger quantities.
- *Leukotrienes* are substances released from the membranes of mast cells during IgE-mediated reactions that cause the uncomfortable bronchoconstriction and excessive secretion of mucus.
- *Antibodies* are specific types of proteins, called immunoglobulins, that are part of the body's defense mechanism. They are made to neutralize a foreign protein in the body.
- *Allergens* are substances that trigger the body's allergic reaction. When the IgE on a mast cell combines with an allergen, an allergic reaction may result.

are introduced later, children have a greater risk of developing allergies to animal dander.

Of course, the hygiene hypothesis requires a great deal more investigation, but it is intriguing that there has been a rise in the rates of allergy and asthma that is consistent with the rise in antiseptic and airtight homes. Time will tell!

Seasonal or Perennial?

Allergic rhinitis takes two different forms, seasonal and perennial. When the symptoms occur because of tree pollen in the spring, grasses in the summer, and weeds in the early fall, they are said to be seasonal. About 20 percent of all Americans suffer from seasonal allergic rhinitis. Year-round allergic rhinitis is considered perennial, and more and more Americans are suffering from it. This type of rhinitis may be triggered by allergy to environmental pollution, dust mites, animal dander, or mold spores or mildew.

Seasonal allergic rhinitis is much easier to treat because the symptoms are short-term. Perennial allergic rhinitis from year-round exposure is more difficult to control. If you have both types, you may be prone to recurrent respiratory problems—sinus, throat, and ear infections; chronic fatigue; and even irritability and difficulty concentrating.

Nonallergic Rhinitis

This type of rhinitis does not occur because of an allergic reaction. Rather, the symptoms of nasal or chest congestion and overproduction of mucus are triggered by cigarette smoke and other pollutants. Strong odors, alcoholic beverages, and cold air or iced drinks can trigger nonallergic rhinitis.

Rhinosinusitis

Rhinosinusitis, the more accurate term for what is commonly termed sinusitis, affects more than 10 percent of the U.S. population. Because the mucous membranes of the nose and sinuses are adjoining and subject to the same disease processes and symptoms of nasal obstruction and drainage, sinusitis without rhinitis is rare.

Chronic rhinosinusitis costs about $5.6 billion a year—and that doesn't include an estimated $70 million annually in lost workdays, as well as a diminished quality of life. It's also necessary to count the 300,000-plus sinus surgeries done annually— many of which would have been unnecessary if prevention and treatment measures had been used early on in the disease.

While uncomplicated viral rhinosinusitis usually resolves in seven to ten days, untreated patients with acute bacterial sinusitis are at risk for developing chronic sinus disease or chronic rhinosinusitis, one of the most common chronic illnesses in the United States. Its symptoms include persistent stuffy nose, thick mucus production, tooth discomfort, facial pain or pressure that worsens with bending forward, and loss of smell.

Though chronic rhinosinusitis causes significant discomfort and health problems, it is not well understood. It is characterized by chronic inflammation with a predominance of eosinophils and T lymphocytes in the tissues, especially in patients with asthma or allergic rhinitis. Viruses, bacteria, and allergic reactions all have been researched and debated as potential mechanisms driving the responses. The immune system mounts different kinds of responses for different invaders—a bacterium gets attacked by a different cell or system than an allergy-prompting particle does, for example. That's why it's critical to identify the key mechanisms in the immune response to chronic rhinosinusitis, allowing researchers to design treatments to relieve the distressing symptoms.

Identifying Allergens

By performing a physical examination, taking your medical history, and doing a series of skin tests to see which allergens react with your system, your doctor can begin to find out the exact substances you are allergic to—or whether you have no allergies at all. Sometimes your keen observation of what causes your symptoms (such as cold air, foods, dust, perfumes, plants, or animals) can help suggest which allergens are responsible for the reactions you feel.

It is also helpful to time your symptoms according to the pollen count published in your newspaper, on TV, or the Internet (see www.pollen.com). For example, if your symptoms start when the ragweed count starts climbing, then stop when ragweed season is over, the chances are great that you are sensitive to ragweed pollen.

Treating Allergic Rhinitis

Whatever type of allergic rhinitis you have, it's important to seek treatment. If left untreated, sinus infections, ear infections, asthma, or a worsening of asthma can result. In fact, sinus infections contribute significantly to the frequency and severity of asthma attacks. You may also get symptoms such as headaches,

Common Outdoor Allergens

- Dust
- Environmental pollution
- Grass
- Industrial pollution
- Mold spores
- Pollen
- Ragweed
- Trees
- Weather changes (cold air, fronts, wind, humidity)

Common Indoor Allergens

- Aerosols
- Certain foods
- Cockroaches
- Cosmetics
- Chemically treated wood and rugs (formaldehyde)
- Dander from pets
- Dust mites
- Feathers
- Fumes
- Mold
- Room deodorizer sprays or vapors
- Smoke
- Wood-burning stove
- Wool

Common Allergens, Irritants, and Physical Changes That Trigger the Allergic Response

- Plant pollens
- Tree pollens (spring)
- Grass pollens (summer)
- Molds and mildew
- Household dust (dust mites)
- Animal dander
- Industrial chemicals
- Cockroaches
- Feathers
- Foods (chocolate, shellfish, milk, citrus, eggs, nuts, corn)
- Food additives or colorings (sulfites or preservatives)
- Medications (aspirin, anti-inflammatory drugs, penicillin, beta-blockers)
- Insect stings
- Hormones
- Smoke
- Perfumes or inhalants
- Respiratory infections
- Gases
- Weather changes
- Cold air
- Exercise

fatigue, and sleep disturbance in the long term with out-of-control allergies.

In most allergic reactions, medications such as antihistamines are prescribed by your doctor (see chapter 10) to counteract the release of histamine. Decongestants are given to help reduce swelling in the nasal passages. If the reaction is severe, you may need steroids—oral, inhaled, or by injection—to reduce swelling. If the inflammation occurs in the bronchial tubes, oral or inhaled bronchodilators are given to help decrease swelling and allow easier breathing.

Pregnancy and Your Nose

About one-half of all pregnant women have symptoms of rhinitis, both allergic and nonallergic, during gestation. This is caused by increased blood volume during pregnancy, progesterone's relaxing effects on nasal blood vessels, and estrogen's tendency to increase swelling of the membrane lining the nose. Nasal congestion will be worse during the second and third trimesters. Nasal polyps, sinusitis, and infectious rhinitis may be worsened due to the factors mentioned. Sinusitis occurs in about 1.5 percent of pregnant women, a rate six times that of the general nonpregnant population. These problems can be so severe as to disturb sleep.

Treatment of nasal symptoms requires precise diagnosis, avoidance measures, and limited medications. Talk to your doctor if you are pregnant and need recommendations for breathing clearly.

ANATOMICAL AND STRUCTURAL PROBLEMS

When your nose is not aligned properly, or there are crevices or projectiles that are not supposed to be there, sinus infections can result.

The nasal septum is the part of the nose that divides the right nasal cavity from the left nasal cavity. When a deviated nasal septum occurs, either from injury or due to a congenital defect, the cartilage and bone in the center of the nose are shifted to one side. This problem keeps mucus from draining properly, leading to the perfect breeding ground for bacteria.

Other anatomical problems can lead to chronic sinusitis. If these problems are severe enough, they may warrant a surgical procedure as well. For example, a septal spur (a sharp projection) causes abnormal secretions due to irritation. A septal perforation (hole) will cause crusting. Deformed or enlarged nasal turbinates (see pages 267–268) can cause blockage of mucus, leading to infections. All of these problems can be corrected with sinus surgery.

Nasal polyps, grape-like growths inside the nasal cavity, affect from 1 to 4 percent of the population; their cause remains unknown. It is thought that polyps form because of excessive growth of the mucous lining in the nose, especially from one of the turbinates. This excessive growth may occur because of chronic allergies or infectious rhinitis. Nasal polyps create even more barriers to sinus drainage, trapping mucus and creating a breeding ground for bacteria. They can also affect your sense of smell.

Nasal polyps normally act like balloons filled with water. When they are healthy, there are tiny holes that let fluid out of the polyps (or balloons). Yet, for some reason, when sinus problems occur, these holes close and the mucus keeps accumulating within the cells like a balloon filling with water.

Although polyps in the cervix or colon are worrisome, nasal polyps are not likely to become malignant and do not have to be removed for biopsy. If the polyps do not block your nose or sinus, most doctors are content to leave them alone.

Polyps can be of allergic origin but usually aren't. They can also result from an aspirin sensitivity (see below). The bottom line is that science is not 100 percent sure what causes nasal polyps.

If you have nasal polyps, your doctor will probably give you a short course of oral corticosteroids combined with an antibiotic (see page 246). The antibiotic is necessary because polyps, by their size and position, block the sinus and nose and form a perfect place for bacteria to breed. (If you put a sterile piece of cotton into your nose for sixteen hours, bacteria will grow because of the blockage; polyps work the same way.) Sometimes the response to the medications is insufficient, and the medication needs to be repeated. Your doctor may prescribe one of the newer steroid nasal sprays, described in chapter 10 (Step 7), to keep the polyps from returning.

If surgery for nasal polyps is necessary, your doctor will order a computed tomography (CT) scan to see how much polypoid tissue is in the sinuses. (*Polypoid* basically means "having polyps.") The good news is that many people with nasal polyps can be successfully treated with medication alone. The bad news is that no matter how successful the medical or surgical treatment is, polyps are notorious for returning. Polyps can return if you take aspirin or salicylates, or if you have a secondary nasal infection. Exposure to dust can precipitate the return of nasal polyps.

ENVIRONMENTAL IRRITANTS

Air pollution, smoke, chemical irritants, weather changes, and even the family pet can cause inflammation and swelling of the narrow channels from the nose to the sinuses. Something as simple as a trip to your local mall during the holidays may set you up for infection if the fragrances pumped into the mall's air trigger sinus inflammation. Again, when a blockage occurs, it leads to poor mucus drainage, bacterial growth, and a resulting sinus infection.

FAMILY HISTORY

"Like parent, like child" may hold true for sinusitis. If one of your biological family members suffers from sinus disease, your own risk increases. The exact reason is unknown, but if both parents have asthma, the probability of having an allergic child is quite high.

IMMUNODEFICIENCY

If you have an impaired immune system, this puts you at a higher risk for sinusitis. The immune system is your body's natural defense system against infection and disease. Its main function is to distinguish self (you) from nonself (a host of invaders) through a complex network of antibodies, proteins, and specialized cells. Your spleen and thymus are crucial organs and produce white blood cells called lymphocytes. These lymphocytes are a type of leukocyte (or white blood cell) that includes natural killer (NK) cells, macrophages, and lymphocytes (B cells and T cells). All of these cells have a mission—to keep you healthy at all costs by attacking and destroying foreign materials.

Lymphocytes act like your personal bodyguards, traveling throughout the body to keep an eye open for any foreign invader. Corresponding troops in the lymph nodes and spleen stay on red alert, ready to go to war at a moment's notice.

Perhaps it would help to think of your immune system as a tag team, which deals with a host of invading viruses, bacteria, and cancer cells. When the receptors sense trouble is brewing, they signal to the antibodies and other cells to stop these invaders. Invaders take the form of bacteria, viruses, parasites, and fungi, all of which are called antigens. When something malfunctions and interferes with this communication, the immune system may fail to function as it should, resulting in the development of autoimmune diseases such as arthritis, allergy, asthma, lupus, and multiple sclerosis. If your immune system is depleted, your body is at risk of being overwhelmed by invading bacteria and viruses, resulting in cancer, life-threatening diseases, or chronic diseases such as sinusitis.

EMOTIONAL STRESS

Given that stress is an important factor for the development of disease, daily stressful events may greatly increase your susceptibility to sinusitis. Your stress level, your beliefs, and your emotions influence the lifestyle choices you make, such as whether you smoke or drink, the foods you eat or don't eat, your bedtime, exercise patterns, and a host of other habits. Typically, an unhealthy lifestyle is a direct response to ongoing stress.

Even anxiety can needlessly reinforce sinusitis and worsen the symptoms.

GASTROESOPHAGEAL REFLUX DISEASE (GERD)

New studies are finding that gastroesophageal reflux disease (GERD), whose prominent symptom is usually heartburn, can damage structures other than the esophagus and result in sinus infections and even eroded teeth and gums. With GERD, you have symptoms of thick mucus in the throat, hoarseness, and difficulty in swallowing. Studies show that one-third of all Americans suffer from GERD at least once a month; 10 percent of all Americans experience it weekly or daily. Findings also report that up to 89 percent of those with asthma suffer from heartburn or GERD as well.

GERD generally occurs at night when you are lying down. Normally a valve between the esophagus and the gastric system prevents stomach acids from backing up into the esophagus. In GERD, this valve does not work properly. The stomach acids reflux or back up into the esophagus, causing irritation and inflammation. Sometimes, if the acidic liquids are aspirated, the lungs can also become inflamed and develop a certain type of pneumonia.

Interestingly, if you have asthma and take theophylline (a bronchodilator medication), it may worsen GERD. This is because the bronchodilator effect relaxes the valve between your stomach and esophagus.

Tests used to diagnose GERD start with a medical examination and personal history. Your doctor may request an

Symptoms of GERD

- Bad breath (halitosis) and a bitter taste in the mouth when one awakens
- Excessive thick phlegm, particularly in the morning
- Heartburn
- Chronic throat clearing and tickle in the throat
- Chronic, irritating cough
- A scratchy, sore throat, particularly in the morning
- Chronic hoarseness
- Sensation of a lump in the throat
- Excess mucus production
- Prolonged vocal warm-up, with low or husky voice quality
- Undependable voice—good one day and hoarse and tired the next
- Vocal fatigue after short periods of singing and speaking
- Trouble breathing or laryngospasm (closing off of the airway)
- Regurgitation of food and liquids
- Exacerbation of asthma (asthma is much more difficult to control when complicated by reflux)

esophageal manometry, a test that measures the pressures inside the esophagus and stomach. A twenty-four-hour esophageal pH test may also be used, as it verifies whether stomach acid refluxes to the esophagus. At times, a special type of X-ray might

Steps to Help End GERD

- Elevate the head of your bed about six inches.
- Sleep with two pillows.
- Don't eat after 8:00 P.M.
- Avoid foods that weaken the lower esophageal sphincter, such as chocolate, peppermint, fatty foods, coffee, and alcoholic beverages.
- Avoid citrus foods, tomatoes, and peppers.
- Lose weight.

be necessary to see the esophagus and how it actually functions during swallowing. Your doctor might recommend flexible laryngoscopy, a test that allows him or her to look at the vocal cords to see if there is redness where the acid from the stomach rises to the back of the larynx (an area between the arytenoids). If this area is red and swollen, it signifies acid irritation from GERD. If there is severe irritation of the esophagus—called Barrett's esophagus—the doctor will order a barium swallow and take a direct look at the esophagus. Barrett's esophagus is serious and can be a premalignant condition. We talk more about these tests in Step 1, page 105.

Treatment for GERD includes over-the-counter or prescription medications (such as Zantac, Tagamet, Axid, Pepcid, Prilosec, or Prevacid, which stop the overproduction of stomach acid) along with lifestyle and dietary changes. In some cases, surgery is necessary to correct the problem.

BLOWING YOUR NOSE TOO HARD

When you do get a cold, go easy on blowing your nose. Studies show that blowing your nose vigorously can make your misery last longer by forcing harmful bacteria into the sinuses. The result? Another sinus infection. So while blowing your nose helps to relieve congestion temporarily, find other means of doing this job, such as nasal irrigation with saline solution or antihistamines (see pages 240–242). Or wipe it gently with a clean tissue.

SINUSITIS TRIGGERS: FACTORS THAT EXACERBATE SINUSITIS

Sinusitis Trigger	Examples	Comments
1. Respiratory infections	Viral, bacterial	Are a common cause of sinusitis exacerbation. Bronchial hyperresponsiveness can last as long as two months after an upper respiratory infection.

2. Allergens	Dust mites, domestic animals, pollens, fungal spores	Sinusitis after dust exposure is usually due to mite allergy. Plant-derived pollens are a common cause of hay fever. Airborne fungal spores may be more important allergens than pollens.
3. Environmental factors	Pollution, sulfur dioxide, smog compounds ozone, weather fronts, cold temperatures, high humidity	Sinusitis symptoms are increased during periods of heavy air pollution.
4. Drugs and food additives	Aspirin, NSAIDs, MSG	Aspirin allergy is commonly associated with nasal polyps. Some food additives cause a chemical reaction.

5. Emotional factors	Stress	Chronic stress can lead to poor lifestyle habits, which increase susceptibility to infection.
6. Others	Smoking, perfumes, inhalants, sprays, paints, alcohol	Secondhand smoke is an important cause of sinusitis. Aromas and fumes are common causes of sinus irritation.

No matter what triggers your bouts of sinusitis, there are some proven and positive steps you can take to get back in control and find excellent relief. As you start to understand your disease, you can begin using the easy suggestions in the seven-step program found here.

Chapter 2

SINUSITIS AND COEXISTING PROBLEMS

Sinusitis can be quite exasperating. Not only do the symptoms of nasal obstruction, congestion, and mucus drainage affect your sleep, appetite, and mood, they can keep you from giving your best performance at home and on the job.

Let's take Cindi, age forty-two, as an example. This active preschool teacher and mother of three children has suffered from sinusitis most of her adult life. "Since my freshman year in college, I have lived with sinusitis and chronic postnasal drip to the point where I am irritable most of the time.

"My doctor prescribed medications that stopped the postnasal drip, but they made me extremely drowsy during daytime hours. This makes it hard to control my class of active preschoolers, much less enjoy time with my own children. After taking the sinus medications at night, I fall asleep easily, only to awaken in a few hours feeling as if I've had two cups of strong coffee.

"When I don't take the medications, my mood, energy level, and ability to concentrate are much better. But without medication I cough constantly from the thick postnasal drip. As a mom and teacher, I have to feel my best each day. Not taking the medication is simply not an option, yet the side effects are often unacceptable to me."

As Cindi laments, any process that affects even the smallest part of the respiratory system frequently disrupts all aspects of an active life. For example, you might be a sinus sufferer who is also allergic to dust mites with increased nasal congestion, purulent mucus production, and difficulty being active or sleeping soundly. The increased resistance to your airflow causes breathing discomfort. Then the subsequent postnasal drip can trigger coughing and even snoring, which adds to your sleep problems and makes you drag through the next day. Similarly, add problems such as asthma to sinusitis and you have even more mucus production, inflammation in the airways, coughing, wheezing, and bronchoconstriction.

Many sinus sufferers have coexisting problems. Some are annoying, such as postnasal drip or an occasional nosebleed, while others are much more serious, such as asthma or blocked ears. Some coexisting problems even confuse the diagnosis of sinusitis!

In this chapter, we'll introduce you to some of these common problems that often occur with sinusitis. We will show you how they are related to sinus disease, and then give you some doctor's recommendations to consider to reduce the symptoms or even resolve the problem altogether.

NOSEBLEEDS

Most sinus sufferers have nosebleeds, particularly when the constant sinus congestion irritates the lining of the nose. When the

nose is dry and crusted, it may bleed, especially if you go to a dry
or cold area at a high altitude or if it's during the winter months
when the furnace blasts dry heat throughout a house or building.
Sometimes the medications used to treat sinusitis, such as the
inhaled nasal steroids or over-the-counter decongestant sprays,
can cause nosebleeds. While a nosebleed looks frightening and
feels bad, in most cases it is not serious.

If you have frequent nosebleeds, it could be a warning sign
of high blood pressure. Talk to your doctor for an accurate diagnosis and treatment.

Doctor's Rx for Nosebleeds

For the sudden or acute nosebleed, try over-the-counter decongestant nasal drops (or spray) such as Neo-Synephrine. Place
the drops (or spray) on a piece of clean cotton and then gently
insert the cotton in your nose, pressing gently from the outside
of the nose. The decongestant is an excellent vasoconstrictor
and will close the blood vessels. (It is best to sit up while doing
this procedure.)

Putting a cold compress (ice pack) to the nose may also
help. Press the coldest part against the upper lip. Most important, stay calm. The more the excited you get, the higher your
blood pressure will rise, resulting in increased bleeding.

For chronic nosebleeds, use saline nose spray (without additives) and an antibiotic ointment such as Neosporin or Baci-
tracin. If the tube has a pointed tip, you can insert it into the soft
part of the nose. Squeeze out a dab of ointment, and then press
on the nose from the outside to spread the ointment around. Do
this two or three times daily. If the tube does not have a tip, put
a pea-sized amount of ointment into the nose with your finger

and press from the outside to spread this around. In many cases of nosebleed, the nose is infected, and the antibiotic ointment helps to resolve the infection—thus the nosebleed will subside.

If you are taking aspirin or aspirin substitutes, including nonsteroidal anti-inflammatory drugs (NSAIDs), this may cause your nose to bleed. Taking the herb ginkgo biloba with aspirin is also a common cause of nosebleeds.

Dry climates are another frequent cause of nosebleeds. If you live in a dry climate, use a saline spray throughout the day to keep the mucosal membrane moist. To keep your bedroom moist at night, use a humidifier or simply hang a wet towel over a chair—both will help increase humidity in the room.

If you have generally fragile blood vessels, your doctor may suggest taking rutin by mouth daily. Rutin, a bioflavonoid extract of lemon peel, is often recommended to strengthen capillaries and stop bruising. You can purchase rutin at most natural food stores. Always talk to your doctor before taking any natural dietary supplement.

POSTNASAL DRIP

Almost everyone has experienced an occasional problem with postnasal drip from time to time. Nevertheless, for many people, debilitating problems such as throat clearing, sore throat, laryngitis, coughing, and even wheezing or asthma symptoms are relentless.

Postnasal drip is an unscientific term that refers to the sensation of thick phlegm in the throat, which can become infected. Your glands in the nose and throat produce mucus continuously (one to two pints per day). This mucus moistens and cleans your nasal membranes, helps warm the air you breathe, and traps inhaled foreign matter. Mucus also helps to fight infection.

In normal situations, the throat is moistened by the secretions from the nasal and throat mucous glands. This is part of the mucous-nasal cilia system that defends us from disease. When the amount of liquid secreted by the nose and sinus is reduced and the cilia of the nose and sinus slow down, the fluid thickens and you become aware of its presence. Because the thick phlegm is unpleasant and often infected because it is not moving, our bodies naturally try to get rid of it.

There are other causes of postnasal drip. For example, at nighttime, many sinus sufferers breathe through their mouths and do not swallow or clear the mucus from their nose. This causes the mucus drainage (postnasal drip) to pool in the back of the throat and nose, creating irritation. Many postnasal drip sufferers tell of feeling the sensation of a lump (called *globus sensation*) in the throat when they swallow, and it causes them to noisily clear their throat or cough repeatedly to relieve it. That is why mornings are particularly difficult for those with chronic sinusitis or nasal allergies.

With age, the swallowing muscles lose strength and coordination. Whereas secretions flowed actively in younger years, older adults may find that they have to clear their throat frequently. Also, many people experience irritation of the throat when under stress. In this situation, the throat muscles tighten or spasm, causing frequent throat clearing.

Doctor's Rx for Postnasal Drip

In order to treat postnasal drip, one must bring the mucous-cilia system back to normal. Nasal irrigation is an excellent solution

Causes of Thin, Clear Mucus

- Colds or flu
- Allergies in the early stage
- Cold temperatures
- Iced drinks
- Certain foods or spices
- Hormonal changes
- Pregnancy
- Bright lights
- Anatomical problems
- Medications
- Vasomotor rhinitis

Causes of Thick, Sticky Secretions

- Too little moisture due to heating of home or office
- Sinus infection
- Allergies in the late stage
- Dairy or food allergies
- Obstruction in nose

Causes of Decreased Secretions

- Exposure to environmental irritants (smoke, pollutants, chemicals, fumes)
- Age (mucous membranes dry and shrink as we get older)
- Structural abnormalities (deviated septum)

for unhealthy cilia, as discussed in chapter 5, and helps to thin the mucus. When mucus is thin, you do not feel it in the back of your throat. Follow the other recommendations in the seven-step program to keep the cilia healthy and mucus thin, such as drinking hot tea throughout the day and avoiding iced drinks.

RHINITIS CAUSED BY MEDICATION

Rhinitis caused by medication (rhinitis medicamentosa) results from chemical irritation when over-the-counter decongestant nasal drops or sprays are used for a prolonged period. These sprays relieve nasal congestion in just minutes by reducing the blood flow to the lining of the nose. However, as the package label explains, you should use these nasal drops or sprays for only three to five days to avoid worsening the inflammation of the lining of the nasal passages and destroying nasal cilia.

If used for more than the recommended time, the nose will become more congested than it was initially because of a rebound effect. As an example, let's ay that you use a nasal spray in the morning and then again twe e hours later. You might experience good relief from your sinusitis or rhinitis for twenty-four hours on this day. Then, invariably, on day two your nose clogs up again, so you use the nasal spray as a decongestant. While you once again feel great relief, you might now find that you need the spray again—but in eight hours—not twelve. On the third day, you might find you need it every six hours—then every four hours on subsequent days. Using the nasal spray more frequently will cause a rebound effect that leads you to use it even more. These medications can cause you to feel nervous and irritable, and also increase the heart rate and disturb sound sleep because of the adrenergic effect of the medication.

There is now evidence that benzalkonium (BZK), a preservative in these decongestant sprays, is the trigger of this rebound inflammation. Products without BZK may not cause rebound rhinitis and congestion, but unfortunately they are available only from a compounding pharmacy and are quite expensive.

Doctor's Rx for Rhinitis Caused by Medication

There are several medical solutions to resolving this uncomfortable condition. One solution is a course of oral prednisone with an antibiotic. This combination of medications will shrink the nasal tissues and reduce inflammation. Also, taking the over-the-counter antihistamine diphenhydramine (Benadryl) at night can help with sleep if your constant congestion is keeping you from getting rest.

Another solution is to gradually dilute the amount of nasal spray (or drops) you are using. For example, take the nasal spray solution and add an equal amount of saline. You can use an over-the-counter saline solution or make your own by adding ½ teaspoon salt to 1 cup warm water. Label this new solution bottle "A." Shake the new solution, and then use bottle A for one week. The next week, add an equal amount of saline and solution from bottle A and label this bottle "B." Use this diluted spray for a week. The third week, remove ½ ounce of the diluted solution from bottle B, and add it to a new bottle labeled "C" along with an equal amount of saline solution. Following this technique of dilution, continue to dilute your nose spray each subsequent week until you no longer have the need to use the spray. You will not experience a rebound effect using

---

Commonly Used Nasal Sprays That Contain Benzalkonium

Brand Name	Generic Name
Afrin	Oxymetazoline
Neo-Synephrine	Phenylepherine
Otrivin	Xylometazoline

---

this simple method of withdrawal, and no medications are necessary.

VASOMOTOR RHINITIS

If you've been to the allergist and all your tests are negative yet you continue to have trouble breathing through your nose, you may have what's called vasomotor rhinitis. With this problem, your nose feels blocked and swollen. You are bothered by postnasal drip and nasal discharge but have no fever. It is difficult to sleep because you cannot breathe through your nose, yet you don't have allergies or sinusitis. Also, the blood IgE level (related to allergy) is normal.

Vasomotor rhinitis or VMR is essentially a nerve imbalance. The internal nose is supplied by a very complex system of nerves that controls liquid production including how much blood flows to the nasal tissues. When more blood flows, the nasal tissues are swollen and there is liquid drainage. One set of nerves enlarges the nasal tissue, and the other set shrinks it.

We don't know why the nerves stop functioning normally. With VMR, finding the right treatment is difficult, as nasal irrigation, dustproofing, change of job or climate, and even relaxation seldom work to treat the problem. Antihistamines seldom work either, and decongestants may give relief but only temporarily.

Doctor's Rx for Vasomotor Rhinitis

What does help vasomotor rhinitis is Atrovent nasal spray because it affects the nerve function. Astelin has been reported to work, too. In difficult cases, your doctor might suggest surgery to alleviate the symptoms.

LARYNGITIS

Laryngitis is hoarseness or loss of voice; it coexists frequently with sinusitis. It is usually caused by inflammation of the moist skin that surrounds the voice box and surrounding tissues, although sometimes thick mucus draining down your throat can cause hoarseness.

With laryngitis, you may have

- A raspy voice
- A dry cough
- A viral infection such as croup
- An irritated or scratchy throat
- A tickle or lump in your throat upon swallowing
- A fever and general malaise
- A bacterial infection

Acute or sudden laryngitis is a common condition that usually occurs with a viral upper respiratory tract infection or vocal strain (yelling, cheering). If the hoarseness is part of a respiratory tract infection, you may have persistent drainage, cough, and mild sore throat. A cough is also commonly associated with laryngitis. The cough could be the result of sinusitis with post-nasal drip, asthma, or gastroesophageal reflux disease (GERD—see pages 34–36). Resolving the associated problem will resolve the cough and hoarseness.

Doctor's Rx for Laryngitis

To resolve laryngitis, stop talking. Don't even whisper. If you need to, use a paper and pencil to express yourself until the voice recovers. Also avoid gargling. While many people believe in gargling with warm salt water to stop laryngitis, it does not help—and actually worsens this condition.

You can try breathing steam with your tongue out to enable the moist heat to get to the larynx. If you use this method, be careful not to burn yourself. Most drugstores have specific breathing appliances that produce steam. Ask your druggist about this appliance, and see if this might help your situation.

Sucking on lozenges (any type) helps to keep the throat moist. You might also try lozenges of papaya and pineapple fruit enzymes dissolved in the mouth between the cheek and gum to help reduce inflammation.

If your laryngitis persists for more than two weeks, see your doctor for an evaluation.

SINOBRONCHIAL SYNDROME

Sinobronchial syndrome is a type of sinusitis that results in lower respiratory tract symptoms such as bronchitis or asthma. It is thought that anywhere from 20 to 70 percent of asthmatic adults have coexisting sinus disease. Conversely, 15 to 56 percent of those with allergic rhinitis or sinusitis have evidence of asthma.

The most likely reason for sinus disease felt in your lower airway is a constant drip of various inflammatory and infective secretions from the back of the nose to the back of your throat. This throat irritation may cause bronchial constriction by a reflex transmitted by the nervous system. Or the postnasal drip of inflammatory secretions from the upper airway may create a secondary inflammatory reaction of the lungs, causing either bronchitis or asthma.

If you have sinobronchial syndrome, you will feel a host of miserable symptoms including shortness of breath, wheezing, productive cough, nasal obstruction, fever, headache, and chest tightness. You may have trouble sleeping because lying down causes an increase in the postnasal drainage and an increase in cough. While some people may have only mild symptoms such as a cough or chest tightness, others have more severe symptoms, which cause them respiratory distress.

With sinobronchitis, you might suffer from sinus inflammation or infection with tenderness over the sinuses, along with constant nasal and sinus drainage. You may also have a rapid respiratory rate, rapid heart rate, and fever. Your lungs can reveal wheezes or rhonchi, which suggest airway inflammation and the presence of mucus. *Rhonchi* are whistling or snoring sounds heard through the stethoscope when listening to the chest.

They indicate partial obstruction of the airways by mucus or other inflammatory debris such as pus. Also, wheezing occurs when the bronchial tubes are narrowed, and can be heard on expiration (breathing out).

Doctor's Rx for Sinobronchial Syndrome

Studies show that aggressive treatment of sinusitis can decrease sinobronchial syndrome and bronchial hyperresponsiveness. Your doctor will do a complete physical examination, and while a chest X-ray may show some evidence of airway inflammation, most are usually normal. Special pulmonary tests are also used to measure airflow. An X-ray of your sinuses might reveal chronic inflammatory changes in the sinuses and possibly evidence of infection. By treating the sinus disease, you can effectively diminish the severity and occurrence of lower airway problems.

As a side note, when all treatments seem to have failed, simple bed rest replenishes the body's cortisone level and often cures the symptoms of sinusitis and related problems. Also, avoid getting chilled to keep sinus symptoms at bay.

Most Common Causes of Chronic Cough in Nonsmokers

- Postnasal drip syndrome
- Asthma
- Gastroesophageal reflux disease (GERD)
- Slow bronchial cilia

COUGH

Cough is one way the body protects itself from allergens. It helps to remove mucus, fluids, and potential infectious material from the airways. But cough is also one of the most prevalent symptoms of lung disease and stems from many different causes, including sinusitis or inflammation in the sinus cavities, postnasal drip due to rhinitis or inflammation in the nasal passages, chronic rhinitis, or GERD. Asthma is a serious cause of cough that is quite common today. Cough-type asthma has been called hidden asthma or cough-variant asthma and is vastly underdiagnosed and undertreated.

If you have a persistent cough, even with no other symptoms such as sinusitis, talk to your doctor. It is helpful to let your doctor know how long the cough has been present, whether any activities or exposures seem to make it worse, if you notice any other different or unusual feelings, and whether the cough is productive. A cough is productive when it brings up phlegm or mucus and unproductive when it is dry.

Essentially, when the normal cilia action fails to bring up unwanted material from the chest, cough takes over. That's why proper intake of fluids is so important to keep your respiratory tract functioning optimally.

Doctor's Rx for Cough

Determining the cause of chronic cough usually involves eliminating probable causes and trying various treatments. A thorough discussion and physical examination will guide your doctor in ordering tests, such as an X-ray of your chest; spirometry, which is a pulmonary function test that shows how your lungs are functioning; and blood tests. Depending on the outcome of the medical tests, your doctor will prescribe treatment, which may include oral medications and/or inhaled bronchodilators and inhaled corticosteroids. If one treatment does not work, be prepared to try other treatments until your doctor finds the most effective medication with the least side effects.

Antibiotic Overuse Is Making Us Sick

Asthma and sinusitis are increasing in frequency and morbidity, despite the advances made in understanding and treating these conditions. Many experts believe the overuse of antibiotics is to blame for this increased incidence and base this on the following:

- A current theory suggests that with overuse of antibiotics, the normal disease reaction is replaced by a hypersensitivity reaction.
- This theory notes a high incidence of disease in families with upper incomes; these individuals have full access to medical care, cleanliness, and dust-proofing (see the discussion of the Hygiene Hypothesis on page 22).
- The body's immune system is designed to fight parasites and infections. If the antibiotic is administered at the first sign of illness, perhaps the normal immunity does not develop and alternative systems are produced (e.g., asthma, poor resistance to infection).

ASTHMA

Asthma is a chronic lung disease characterized by inflammation, airway obstruction, and hyperresponsiveness.[1] This serious illness often coexists with sinusitis and affects more than 15 million people in the United States. With asthma, your airways are "twitchy" and become inflamed when they meet such stimuli as allergens or cold air. When you have an attack, spasms of the bronchial muscles, along with swelling of the mucous membrane lining the bronchi and excessive amounts of mucus, contribute to airway narrowing. Consequently, the airway resistance and the work of breathing increase to cause wheezing and shortness of breath. You may have a cough due to irritation inside the airway and the body's attempt to clean out the accumulations of mucus.

Why you have airway inflammation and bronchial hyperreactivity and others do not is unclear. Allergy clearly plays an important role in many asthma cases, but not in all. Sinusitis plays a role as well. Like allergy and sinusitis, asthma has a strong genetic component. In some patients, the inflammation of the sinuses and the bronchial system is the same illness (see the section on sinobronchial syndrome, pages 51–52).

Asthma Triggers

Triggers are those elements that cause your asthma attack by initiating airway inflammation and bronchospasm. Your asthma triggers will not be the same as someone else's and can even vary at different times in your life. However, by identifying those elements that trigger your breathing problems, you can take steps to avoid or limit exposure and have better control of your asthma symptoms.

What You May Feel

While many people have the onset of asthma in early child-hood, first asthma symptoms can occur at any age. Typically, you will experience episodes of cough and shortness of breath with intervals of complete remission. A nonproductive cough and wheeze often accompany the onset of an asthma attack. After a period of time, you may suddenly experience the sensation of suffocation and chest tightness. Still, sometimes the only symptom you have is a dry cough.

The severity of asthma attacks and symptoms varies from time to time and person to person. If you have had asthma for a long time, you may experience chronic cough, wheezing, and decreased stamina during exercise. It is highly common to develop asthma symptoms when laughing, singing, or crying. Many people have a worsening of airflow obstruction at night and in the early morning hours for reasons that are still unclear.

Individuals with asthma often have a lengthy childhood history of allergy and suffer with chronic wheezing, coughing, and sleepless nights. Also associated with these symptoms are frequent sinus infections with heavy pus or thick mucus drainage into the chest. Whenever individuals with asthma get a sinus infection, the asthma worsens and does not clear with simple treatment. When the nose is obstructed, patients tend to breathe with the mouth open, which precipitates an asthma attack. Patients with asthma have a dry mouth all the time and are bothered by thick nasal phlegm dripping into the throat. The thick phlegm causes the patients to cough and clear the throat constantly.

If you look back to a time when you had an asthma attack, usually you will find exposure to some trigger before the onset of symptoms. While the onset of a cough, shortness of breath, and wheezing is gradual in most people, in a few people life-threatening airflow obstruction may develop within a matter of a few hours. This is especially true for about 15 percent of those with asthma who are not aware of the degree of the severity of their airway obstruction. Frequently, these people rush to the emergency room with severe airflow obstruction. They are at a higher risk of asthma-related complications, such as need for mechanical ventilation, air leaks from the lung (pneumothorax), and even death.

Anxiety and Asthma

An asthma attack always causes anxiety, especially in a young child. That's why it might help to practice a form of relaxation that can be used when an asthma attack is impending. By reducing the anxiety associated with the attack, the asthma attack can be shortened and the medications may be more effective.

Stand before a mirror so you can see your face and chest. Breathe in to the count of four, and breathe out to the count of six. Make sure your exhalation is longer than your inhalation. Notice how your shoulders relax as you exhale. Your face, forehead, and jaw should also relax. Let the exhalation be a signal to relax your muscles. By practicing this before an asthma attack, you can then use it to possibly avert an attack. Children benefit from learning this procedure, too.

Diagnosing Asthma

Asthma is tough to diagnose during a physical examination. In a normal asthma attack, wheezing and hyperinflation of the chest usually happen. But often by the time you get to the doctor's office, these symptoms are gone. Although you might have a normal chest X-ray, this does not rule out asthma. While your breathing may be normal at the doctor's office, a one-time measurement does not reflect the severity of airflow obstruction during an actual asthma attack. Nasal polyps may be a clue to asthma if you have aspirin-induced bronchospasm (page 74). The best test to measure how well you can breathe is spirometry or peak flow metering. This test measures how much air you can exhale and is the most accurate pulmonary function test used in confirming asthma.

Aspirin Sensitivity, Asthma, and Nasal Polyps

Some people cannot take aspirin or nonsteroidal anti-inflammatory drugs (NSAIDs) because of the aspirin/nasal polyp triad. This aspirin sensitivity occurs in about 10 to 15 percent of people with asthma and 30 to 40 percent of those who have asthma and nasal polyps. You might feel such symptoms as itching, rashes, hives, swelling, nasal congestion, and wheezing after taking a nonsteroidal anti-inflammatory drug. Talk to your doctor about alternative therapies if you have this sensitivity.

Warning Signs and Symptoms of Asthma

- Increased frequency of wheezing and dyspnea
- Decreasing ability to exercise
- Cough productive of sputum, which is getting thicker
- Shortness of breath
- Restlessness
- Wheezing or coughing, especially at night or after exercise
- Feeling of tightness in the chest
- Worsened sleep quality because of wheezing or attacks of breathlessness
- More frequent use of bronchodilator drugs
- Fast breathing (hyperventilation)

Doctor's Rx for Asthma

Treatment for asthma varies from simply avoiding asthma triggers to combinations of smooth muscle relaxants, bronchodilators, and anti-inflammatory medications. Because asthma is considered an inflammatory condition, antibiotics may be required as well.

SNORING

Snoring commonly exists with acute or chronic sinusitis, because of changes in the upper airway from the back of the nose to the base of the tongue that occur during sleep. The muscles supporting the opening of the upper airway relax during sleep, and extra tissue in the palate and uvula—the fleshy piece between the tonsils—vibrates with each breath. There is a tendency for the airway to close at any point along this pathway.

Snoring or Obstructive Sleep Apnea?

An old wives' tale has suggested that primitive men defended their women at night by making horrible sounds to scare off predators. We now know that snoring may be an early warning sign for various medical problems, especially for obstructive sleep apnea (OSA). While snoring is caused by the vibration of

---

Common Risk Factors for Snoring

- Sleeping on your back
- Overweight, especially fat stores in the neck
- Cigarette smoking and heavy alcohol drinking
- Allergy, sinusitis, or asthma
- Facial shape
- Narrowed airways due to nasal obstruction, deviated septum, or polyps

---

> ## Conditions That May Result from Snoring with Obstructive Sleep Apnea
>
> - Hypertension, arrhythmias, heart disease, stroke, and even brain damage
> - Personality changes, irritability, and hormonal imbalances
> - Impotence and morning headaches
> - Night sweats, heartburn, or nerve damage
> - Sinusitis, bronchitis, lung disease, and some stomach diseases

the soft parts of the throat while breathing during sleep, the noise may be continuous with almost every breath, or it may be intermittent, with breath-holding spells. These periods of suspension of breathing are called *apneas*, which are due to obstruction of the upper airway at the level of the uvula or base of the tongue. Apneas may be recorded in a sleep disorder laboratory by brain waves and oxygen levels.

Those with OSA not only snore but have other symptoms including:

- Headaches
- High blood pressure
- Dry mouth
- Sore throat upon awakening
- Depression

■ Concentration problems
■ Daytime sleepiness and fatigue

This disorder is found in 20 to 30 percent of those with hypertension. It is also found in those who have sinusitis, nasal blockages or obstructions, enlargement of the tonsils or adenoids, or a misplaced jawbone.

Getting an Accurate Diagnosis

While more than 55 percent of those who snore never even discuss this with their physician, getting an accurate diagnosis is important in order to determine if you have OSA. If you snore and have one or more of the common symptoms, your primary care physician may refer you to a sleep clinic, where you will be evaluated by a sleep disorder specialist. This is a physician (usually a pulmonologist, neurologist, psychiatrist, or sometimes otolaryngologist) who has done additional training and obtained experience in this area in order to pass a special qualifying examination for certification by the American Board of Sleep Medicine.

Doctor's Rx for Snoring and OSA

Although there are different treatments for snoring and for OSA, both surgical and nonsurgical, the best way to guarantee that the treatments will work is to lose weight, if you are over a normal weight. In fact, gaining weight after having surgery for sleep apnea can worsen the problem.

While some people may respond to an orthodontic device that brings the jaw forward at night, there are also office procedures your doctor can perform that are safe and effective. For an office procedure, your doctor does not have to worry about taking away too much tissue the first time; the patient can always return for a second try if needed. This is why office procedures are more desirable for doctor as well as patient.

Radio-frequency ablation (such as somnoplasty) is a commonly used office method to reduce snoring. The doctor first determines which area is vibrating loudly. Then specially placed needles are used to conduct radio-frequency energy into the area under the skin of the palate. The current will cause scarring and atrophy while leaving the skin of the palate unharmed.

Another office method involves injecting sclerosing solution into the soft palate. The sclerosing solution scars and stiffens the palatal tissue, often leaving the skin intact. Still another commonly used procedure is the pillar method. Under local anesthesia in the doctor's office, three rods (similar to collar stays) are inserted in such a way that they keep the soft palate from vibrating and falling back.

Other suggestions to resolve snoring include using over-the-counter Breathe Right nasal strips to open up the nose; keeping the inside of the nose moistened; elevating the head of the bed or trying to sleep on two pillows; and, because snoring is worse when lying on the back, sewing a tennis ball into a cloth pocket in the back of a T-shirt and wearing this during sleep.

The most effective treatment for OSA is continuous positive airway pressure (CPAP). This is a custom-fitted nasal mask that you wear during sleep. This mask is attached to a quietly functioning pump, which delivers air into the airway to prevent it from collapsing. CPAP is successful in almost 90 percent of cases, helping to improve sleep quality and alleviate daytime drowsiness, as well as other serious symptoms. It acts as a support to prevent further narrowing or collapse of your airway, and it actually increases the size of the airway behind the palate and at the back of your tongue. Nasal CPAP not only relieves the symptom of excessive daytime sleepiness but has also been shown to be effective in improving and reducing the severity of medical problems associated with sleep apnea. You may experience such minor side effects as drying of the nasal membrane, nasal congestion, or skin abrasion on the bridge of the nose, but your doctor will help you reduce these effects.

Other more complicated surgical procedures include surgery to remove vibrating or obstructive tissue, surgery to move the tongue forward, and surgical correction of nasal obstructive conditions. For instance, uvulopalatopharyngoplasty (UPPP) removes obstructive tissue, including the tonsils, to open the airway and help to alleviate snoring. Genioglossus and hyoid advancement moves the tongue and laryngeal structures forward to open the airway.

In children it is enlarged adenoids that most often causes snoring or sleep apnea.

DIZZINESS AND VERTIGO

Sometimes when your sinuses are congested, you may experience feelings of dizziness. Dizziness is a feeling of imbalance or disequilibrium, yet you do not feel the sensation of spinning. You may feel unsteady, faint, or have difficulty in walking. Vertigo, another term people use to describe feeling off-balance, is different—it is the sensation of moving, turning, or spinning.

Either you feel like you are moving, or the room feels like it is moving. This often occurs when the fluid in the inner ear is affected.

Motion sickness is another phenomenon people associate with dizziness. You may have experienced this while driving in a car, riding in a plane or boat, or on a spinning ride at the amusement park. While not a serious disorder, motion sickness can make you feel like something is horribly wrong, as your entire body is affected.

The causes of dizziness vary, including the following:

- *Poor blood circulation.* Blood circulation disorders are the most common causes of dizziness. For example, if you feel dizzy from getting up out of bed too fast, it's probably because the blood hasn't had a chance to catch up with your brain. Or when any part of the balance circuit is not getting enough blood, you will feel dizzy or faint. Some people are light-headed because of poor circulation or as a result of hypertension, diabetes, or hardening of the arteries. Anemia is still another cause of lack of blood flow to the brain resulting in dizziness, and stimulants (caffeine, nicotine, other drugs) can also decrease blood flow.
- *Injuries.* A blow to the head, even severe whiplash, can cause some swelling in the circuits and make balancing a problem. Anytime the inner ear is injured, it can result in vertigo with subsequent loss of hearing and nausea.
- *Infections.* A viral or bacterial infection can "attack" your inner ear, resulting in dizziness or vertigo. Mas-

toiditis, a serious infection that extends far into your inner ear, can destroy your hearing and equilibrium.

■ *Allergies*. If you suffer from allergies along with sinus problems, whenever you are exposed to an irritant (pollen, dust mites, mold, food, animal dander, chemicals, etc.) the chances are great that you may have dizziness. As the mucus produced from the allergic reaction subsides, usually the dizziness will go away.

■ *Diseases*. Any neurological disease that affects your balance can result in dizziness or vertigo.

Doctor's Rx for Dizziness

Your doctor will ask how long you have felt the dizziness, how long it lasts, when you feel it most, and what seems to trigger it. After doing a thorough physical examination, your doctor may perform one of the tests discussed in chapter 4. In some cases, your doctor may do blood tests or evaluate your heart if other causes of dizziness are suspected. Hearing tests are recommended for those who have suffered hearing loss.

There are different treatments for dizziness or vertigo, and most depend on specific lifestyle strategies:

■ Refrain from moving your head rapidly.

■ Move slowly when you change positions in bed or while sitting down.

■ Avoid products that are known triggers for your allergies to keep allergic reactions at bay.

■ If you have mucus buildup from sinusitis, ask your doctor for a decongestant to help the sinuses drain.

Grab a Paper Bag to Stop Dizziness

If you are breathing rapidly through your mouth, you may give off too much carbon dioxide (CO_2). This will make you feel light-headed or dizzy. A quick remedy for this is to blow in a paper bag. This helps to restore proper CO_2 levels in the body.

- Keep mucus thin by drinking 8 to 10 cups of water per day. You may also try an expectorant such as guaifenesin (page 254), which is available over the counter in pill form (Mucinex).
- Try taking papaya enzyme. For this, swallow the pill instead of using it buccally. This will help to reduce inflammation and thin mucus.
- De-stress, as anxiety is a common cause of dizziness.
- Keep your blood pressure in a normal range if you have hypertension, and do the same with your blood sugar if you are diabetic.

HALITOSIS (BAD BREATH)

Halitosis (bad breath) is an annoying problem that goes hand in hand with sinusitis. Bad or stale-smelling breath is particularly bothersome because you may not know you have it unless someone tells you. Still, bad breath can spoil your social and work life.

When bacteria stagnate, or remain in one place, they multiply and give off toxins and odors. Another common cause of breath problems are the deep holes in the tonsils known as crypts. These holes are supposed to be there—they provide areas where the good white cells of the body can fight the bad bacteria. The dead bacteria and dead white cells are then extruded and swallowed. But when the holes in your tonsils get too wide or crooked, a cheese-like substance accumulates and causes odor.

Other causes of bad breath include gum disease or dental problems. Also, gastrointestinal problems can result in stale or bad-smelling breath.

Doctor's Rx for Halitosis

Your doctor will take your medical history and do a thorough physical examination. Of particular importance will be an evaluation of your mouth, teeth, gums, throat, and sinuses. If you have gastrointestinal problems, other tests will be performed to see if you may have an ulcer or GERD (see pages 34–36). Any dental problems will be referred to your dentist for evaluation and treatment.

To treat halitosis, your doctor may recommend the following:

- Use salt water nose spray or pulsating nasal irrigation if you have crusts or other sources of odor.
- Have your dentist check your teeth for cavities or gum disease. Treat accordingly.
- Eat yogurt to replenish the good bacteria. It will promote a healthier mouth.

- Floss regularly to keep gum disease at bay.
- Drink eight glasses of water per day. Your mouth may be extra dry from lack of fluids.
- Take a papaya enzyme tablet to aid digestion (see pages 206–207).
- Use lactase tablets if you are milk-intolerant and suffer with gastrointestinal problems.
- Reduce excess stomach acid with Tagamet or Zantac (both are available over the counter). (It is best not to self-diagnose on hyperacidity in the stomach. See your doctor if this is a concern.)
- See www.earaid.info for suggested products.

TINNITUS

Tinnitus (ringing in the ears) may occur with (or without) chronic sinusitis. This "head noise" affects nearly 38 million Americans and may come and go, or it may be with you continuously. It can vary in pitch from a low whine to a high-pitched squeal and can affect one or both ears. More than 7 million people are unable to live normal lives because of the continuous problem of tinnitus—disrupting sleep, thoughts, and work.

In some cases, tinnitus is caused by Menière's disease, an increase in fluid pressure in the inner ear. High or low blood pressure, diabetes, aging, thyroid problems, or tumors may also cause tinnitus. Loud noises and associated hearing loss are contributing factors to this constant noise, as is earwax. Large doses of aspirin and certain aspirin products may bring it on. Stress is not a cause, but once tinnitus becomes annoying, you definitely will feel stressed.

Doctor's Rx for Tinnitus

It's difficult to diagnose tinnitus because there are no specific laboratory tests that indicate it accurately. Your doctor will take a medical history and do a thorough physical examination. Then using X-rays, laboratory tests, and balancing tests, the diagnosis will be narrowed down. During this exam, your doctor may discover specific causes of tinnitus such as hypertension or earwax. If no cause is determined, you will work with your doctor to find methods of treatment that work.

To treat tinnitus, try the following:

- Take vitamin B_6 (pyridoxine), 100 milligrams twice a day for three months.
- Ask your doctor about muscle biofeedback. You cannot feel anxiety when the muscles are fully relaxed.
- Use the stress management tips in chapter 9 (Step 6) to decrease anxiety and tension.
- Use a masking sound that "covers" the tone of the tinnitus. Whether your tinnitus is the type that can be masked or not can be tested by an audiologist.
- Reduce your blood pressure with lifestyle changes or with medications.
- Balance your blood sugar if you're a diabetic.
- Avoid aspirin and NSAIDs if these medications appear to trigger your tinnitus.

EVERYONE'S SINUS PROBLEM IS DIFFERENT

No matter what problems you have along with sinusitis, each person is different. While this book cannot replace a proper medical diagnosis, it can help you become more informed about sinusitis and possible cures. Once you understand the many causes, symptoms, and coexisting problems of sinusitis, you can knowledgeably seek a professional diagnosis from your doctor and begin treatment that works.

Chapter 3

SINUS PAIN . . . AND WHAT YOU CAN DO TO END IT

I haven't slept through the night in two years because of sinus headaches. As if on cue, I wake up in the middle of the night with a throbbing pain behind my eyes. Then I feel dull and lethargic the next day.

—LEE, *age fifty-four*

In college I was a voice major and performed solos with the university chorale. That was before sinusitis. Now, ten years later, I can't even sing with the radio because of vocal damage from the constant postnasal drip. My throat hurts all the time, and nothing I do seems to help.

—RITA, *age thirty*

Even though I've had sinus surgery, my ears are always filled with fluid. When I swallow, they fill with fluid and I can hardly hear, not to mention the shooting pains. Sometimes when I'm really congested, I lose my balance from dizziness.

—PETER, *age forty-six*

If there is one symptom sinus sufferers have in common, it is *pain*. This pain is felt all over the face—and not just in the "sinus" area. Pain can be felt in the jaw just in front of the ear, or it may be felt over the side of the face and head, then extend to the back of the neck, next to the hairline. Sinus pain is often constant, throbbing, and becomes worse with chewing or bending over.

Pain in the sinus comes from pressure on the membranes. Often the most severe pain comes when a vacuum is formed. For example, if you are flying at a high altitude, your nose may clog because of the dryness in the plane's cabin and your failure to drink adequate fluids, such as hot tea. Your nose closes, and almost immediately your body starts to absorb the oxygen in the sinus, which is now plugged. Upon landing, the sinus is now at a low pressure, whereas the atmosphere outside is at a higher pressure. The resulting pain you feel is comparable to a five-pound weight on your eyes. Scuba divers experience similar situations with the changing pressure.

SINUS HEADACHE—A COMMON PROBLEM

You have great company if you suffer with painful sinus headaches. In fact, surveys report that 70 to 90 percent of women and men experience headaches. Of this number, 40 to 50 percent of women and men report headaches that they consider to be disabling. Headaches can be brief and mild (the most common), or they can be severe and frequent. Headaches can be horrible whether the underlying cause is minor or life-threatening. When the pain is severe, it can be disabling no matter what the cause. But whether the symptoms of your headache are from sinusitis, stress, or PMS (premenstrual syn-

---

Symptoms of a Sinus Headache

- Unending or constant pain over cheek or forehead
- Tenderness over the affected sinus and behind the eyes
- A deep, dull ache
- Pain that worsens with movement of your head, such as bending over
- Nasal blockage and congestion
- Nasal discharge
- Ear sensations or ear pressure
- Facial swelling
- Fever (sometimes)

---

drome), an unusual or especially painful headache *should* be evaluated by your doctor.

What Causes the Pain?

Any allergic reaction or even a tumor in the sinuses can produce swelling and blockage of the sinuses, causing the headache pain you feel. Although not all pain in the sinus area is directly related to sinus disease, some of the most common causes of the pain include:

- *Obstruction*. When the cilia become damaged or do not work effectively, the mucus builds up, causing an obstruction. This obstruction of the sinuses and impacted mucus result in decreased oxygen in your sinus cavities. When the ostia (small openings) in the sinus are blocked, the pressure in your sinus cavity increases, leading to the pain that you feel.

■ *Inflammation*. Sometimes sinus pain is due to extreme swelling of the membranes against a deviated nasal septum or nerve area. Or if you suffer sinus pain while in cold air, you may have a wide nose where the bones don't come together. When the roof of your nose is open, cold air strikes the membranes directly, resulting in excruciating pain.

■ *Referred pain*. Sometimes what you may think is a "sinus headache" is really "referred" pain from the neck. How can you tell? Feel the back of your neck when the headache begins. Does the pain from the back of your neck travel to the front of your forehead? This is because of the hookup of the nerves, which can cause painful stimuli to radiate to the front area above your eyes.

■ *Tension*. Tension headaches (or muscle contraction headaches) are caused by the tightening of the muscles of the neck and head. This is common in times of stress or when you are tired. Tension headaches feel like a dull pain with a tightness, a band, or pressure in or around the head. The pain may extend over the top of the head to the front. Your neck or jaws can have pain if there is tightness of the muscles in these areas, too. Tension headaches occur in both women and men, and it is common for family members to have similar headaches.

■ *Stress*. Stress can also cause pain in the jaw and temples, mimicking sinus pain. This can result in more tension in the muscles of the jaw, temples, face, and neck, which causes more spasm and pain. Clenching the teeth during the day or grinding the teeth at night can result from stress and increase the tension on muscles around the jaw. (See chapter 9 for ways to reduce your stress.)

■ *Vascular headaches*. Vascular headaches are usually caused by enlargement (dilation) of arteries in and around the head, which causes the pain. The most common type is migraine headache. Migraines affect an estimated 10 to 20 million people, or as many as 16 percent of women and 9 percent of men out of the total population. These headaches can last from a few hours up to days, and they are dull, throbbing, constant, and severe. They may happen only occasionally or recur within days. They are most often (but not always) on one side of the head and are usually felt in the front or side of the head. Nausea or vomiting generally accompany the headache, and occasionally you may have diarrhea. Lights and a bright room can make the headache much worse. In some forms of migraine headache (called the "classic migraine"), you may see blind spots, light flashes in your vision, or other visual changes before the start of the headache.

■ *Trigeminal neuralgia*. The trigeminal nerve is the fifth cranial nerve. It is centrally located in origin and provides three divisions for pain:

1. To the frontal area
2. To the maxillary, or cheek, area
3. To the jaw

Trigeminal neuralgia means that all of the face is in pain. The trigeminal nerve can be irritated by a viral infection and cause a type of neuralgia, which mimics a sinus headache.

■ *Arthritis headaches.* Arthritis in the neck can be a cause of headache. The most common type of arthritis in this case would be osteoarthritis (the "wear and tear" type of arthritis). However, rheumatoid arthritis, fibromyalgia, and ankylosing spondylitis may also cause headaches. You may feel pain and tenderness in the muscles of the neck, which can add to your headache pain.

■ *Premenstrual headaches.* These headaches start just before the onset of the menstrual period and are usually caused by weight gain as well as water retention.

■ *TMJ syndrome.* A source of pain in the jaw and nearby areas in the face and neck is temporomandibular joint (TMJ) syndrome. Sometimes TMJ mimics sinus pain, but its cause and treatment are different. TMJ is a common problem, with 12 to 20 percent of adults affected. This condition is common in younger adults and may be less frequent after age fifty. With TMJ you will feel pain in the jaw and neck area, but there may also be a sensation of cracking in the jaw when the mouth is opened. Pain may limit the opening of the jaw. The jaw may move to one side when it is opened as well. Headaches are common, along with jaw pain. (See page 79 for Doctor's Rx.)

■ *Ear infection.* Ear diseases or infection can cause pain that is felt more as jaw pain than ear pain, even though the problem is in the ear. Sometimes the pain in the ear is so real that cotton swabs or other objects are used to try to clean the ear. Specific treatment of the ear disease is needed in this case to help the jaw pain, so see a physician.

■ *Other medical problems.* Other types of headaches include those caused by high blood pressure (hypertension) and other medical problems. These can include fever, some chemicals, alcohol use, allergy reaction, and certain foods.

■ *Serious causes of headache.* Problems inside your head can cause headaches, which can be mistaken for sinus headache. A common concern you may have is that there could be a brain tumor. Headaches are the first sign in only a third or less of brain tumors. There are usually other signs your doctor will find upon examination.

■ *Less common causes of headache.* Infections, injuries to the head, inflammation of the nerves and arteries, and diseases of the eye, ear, nose, or teeth are possible causes of headaches, but they are not as common. You may be concerned that your severe headache is a sign of a stroke, but this is a very uncommon cause of chronic headaches.

Since each of these headaches may have treatment options available, it is important to first identify the underlying problem. Talk with your physician to obtain advice.

Doctor's Rx for TMJ

1. Draw a straight vertical line on your mirror.
2. Line up your jaw, mouth, and nose with the straight line.
3. Practice opening your mouth so that your jaw muscles appear balanced on both sides.
4. Now practice relaxing so that the jaw opens automatically in the midline.
5. If you have inflammation or pain, use nonsteroidal anti-inflammatory medicine (Advil or Aleve). Or try Clear•Ease or some other brand of papaya-pineapple buccal enzyme to reduce swelling.

Diagnosing the Headache

In addition to discussing your medical history and giving you a thorough physical examination, your doctor may ask you to have a few tests to help find the cause of the pain. Blood tests, X-rays of the skull or neck, a computed tomography (CT) scan, or magnetic resonance imaging (MRI) may be needed to make a definitive diagnosis.

Treating the Headache

Therapy for sinus headaches is usually directed toward relieving the infection, inflammation, or accompanying allergy. Symptomatic relief includes:

- Taking analgesics such as aspirin, acetaminophen, or nonsteroidal anti-inflammatory drugs (NSAIDs)
- Using nasal vasoconstrictors (over-the-counter decongestant nasal sprays) for a short period
- Trying inhaled nasal corticosteroids (to relieve nasal symptoms with allergy)
- Taking prescribed antibiotics, as listed on page 251, for infections
- Using decongestants to reduce swelling inside the nose
- Taking guaifenesin (the active ingredient in Robitussin or Humabid) to thin thick mucus, making it easier to drain
- Using papaya and bromelain buccal tablets to reduce inflammation

Note: Papaya enzyme tablets are available at most drug or natural food stores. These tablets, taken buccally (held between the cheek and gum), can help to reduce the inflammation associated with sinusitis, nasal congestion, earache, or sore throat. Take one tablet four times a day. (This is especially useful if the pain follows flying or scuba diving.) Clear•Ease is a buccal tablet that contains the anti-inflammatory fruit enzymes papain and bromelain. See chapter 8 for more information on the benefits of papaya enzymes.

Here are some other helpful tips to reduce sinus pain:

- Avoid getting chilled.
- Use warm, moist cloths on the sinus area for ten to fifteen minutes twice a day, to reduce inflammation and pain.
- Breathe in steam, to open the sinuses.
- Stay hydrated by drinking plenty of water daily.
- Drink six to eight cups of hot tea to heal the cilia.
- Use nasal irrigation to remove pus and stimulate natural nasal function.

BACTERIAL SINUS INFECTIONS

Pain resulting from bacterial sinus infections is surprisingly rare, even when X-rays show significant sinus disease. Drainage of the pus is usually done in your doctor's office, particularly localized shrinking and suction of pus and mucus. Your doctor may instruct you on how to use nasal irrigation, as described in chapter 5, at home to continue drainage. He or she also may prescribe antibiotics and decongestants for continued healing. Apply hot compresses over the sinus area and drink hot tea, about six to eight cups a day, to help restore movement to the microscopic cilia of the nose and sinuses.

SORE THROAT PAIN

"It hurts to swallow, and food tastes horrible." Ron's battle with a constantly sore throat was unending. "When I forget to take medication at night, my throat is raw in the morning from post-nasal drip."

A sore throat is a real "pain in the neck," and most people who battle sinus problems know this feeling well! Whether from the constant postnasal drip irritating the delicate tissue, swelling from inflamed tissue, or an all-out throat infection, sore throats hurt and take away from your quality of life and productivity. Sore throat is one of the most common medical complaints, sending nearly 40 million adults to the doctor's office each year for diagnosis and treatment.

To understand why your throat hurts, it's important to know how the throat works. Your throat has three parts:

1. The *nasopharynx*, or part behind the nose at the top of the throat, where the tubes that run from the ears to the nose open.
2. The *oropharynx*, or middle throat, where the tonsils are located.
3. The *laryngopharynx*, or lower part. This is behind and below the tongue, where the larynx, or voice box, is located.

When the top one-third of the throat is affected, your ears may also become infected because the infection travels up the Eustachian tube into the middle ear. When the lower one-third of the throat is infected, you may be hoarse because the larynx is swollen and can't function properly (see pages 49–50). And in fact, many people *get* hoarse because they gargle with warm salt water to try to heal their sore throat! This is like rubbing your eyes when they are infected!

Causes of a Sore Throat

Your nose and throat are constantly defending against outside elements and bacteria. When bacteria settle in the nose, they are seized and dragged off to "battle stations," or lymph glands, where the good white cells are kept. More good blood comes to the area. There the concentration of good white cells can overwhelm the bacteria. But when the lymph material swells, this causes the symptom you feel—a painful throat.

Your throat infection may be from a bacteria or a virus. Or it may be part of a generalized infection. The most important difference between viruses and bacteria is that bacteria respond well to antibiotic treatment, but viruses do not.

Some of the most common causes of sore throat include:

- *Sinus drainage.* If you have constant postnasal drip down the back of your throat or a sinus infection, you may have a sore throat, particularly in the morning. The pain you feel may be caused by breathing through your mouth (and not your nose!) at night and will resolve itself later in the morning. Sometimes an antihistamine taken at night to alleviate allergies can cause a sore throat if the throat becomes dried out.
- *Tonsillitis.* This common throat infection occurs when the tonsils, the lymphatic tissues in the back of the

throat, become infected. In a healthy mouth, the tonsils help to prevent infection in the body by filtering out bacteria and other microorganisms. In some cases, usually when you are run-down and have poor resistance to infection, the tonsils become overwhelmed by viral or bacterial infections. (Chronic tonsillitis can be a source of recurrent infection with strep or *Haemophilus influenzae*.) With tonsillitis, you may have a sore swollen throat and difficulty swallowing because of the inflammation. If you look at your tonsils with a mirror, they will appear red, swollen, and coated in white spots. You may also have a fever and feel fatigued and achy all over.

■ *Gastroesophageal reflux disease* (GERD). GERD, as explained on pages 34–36, is another cause of sore throat. This occurs with the regurgitation of stomach acids into the back of the throat.

■ *Swollen uvula.* The uvula is the part that hangs down the middle of your throat from the soft palate, and a swollen uvula causes a painful throat. The uvula rises up when you swallow, to keep food from going up into the nose. Yet the uvula can swell as an allergic reaction, just as the eyes or nose can. Or sometimes crackers can scratch the uvula and cause swelling. Infection can occur here as well as in the tonsils or the back of the throat, except that swelling of the uvula is quite frightening because of the fear that it will obstruct the airway. It rarely does—but it may feel like it.

■ *Mono* (*infectious mononucleosis*). With mono (commonly called "the kissing disease"), you may feel exhausted and have a fever, very swollen tonsils with a white coating, and an enlarged spleen. A blood test is needed to diagnose mono, and treatment is limited. See your doctor if this is suspected.

■ *Strep* (*streptococcus group* A). The strep bacteria are the cause of sore throat in 20 to 30 percent of cases. Symptoms of strep throat may include fever, red or white spots on the tonsils, swollen and tender neck glands, headaches, nausea, and a fine rash called scarlet fever. See your doctor immediately if you suspect strep throat. This infection usually needs treatment with antibiotics because of rare complications such as rheumatic fever (which can lead to heart damage) or poststreptococcal glomerulonephritis (a kidney complication wherein blood and protein are detected in the urine).

■ *Epiglottitis*. This is the most serious type of throat infection. It's caused by bacteria that target part of the voice box (the larynx), resulting in inflammation or swelling that actually closes the airway. You may have difficulty swallowing or speaking, and breathing will become labored. Emergency medical attention is necessary should this happen.

Diagnosing a Sore Throat

Your doctor will start by taking your medical history. Then, after a thorough physical examination, the throat, tonsils, ears, and sinuses will be checked. Your temperature will be taken to see whether there is fever, and your doctor may take a culture using a dry swab or a rapid strep test (which usually takes a few minutes to do in the office) to see whether you have strep. The lymph glands in your neck will be checked. If they are swollen and tender, it may indicate an acute infection. If they are swollen but not tender, the infection may be chronic, or long-term.

Treating Sore Throat Pain

For sore throat pain:

- Take the full course of antibiotics, as prescribed by your doctor, if needed.
- If the tonsils are "touching," your doctor may prescribe a short course of oral steroids to reduce swelling. Take these as directed.
- Do not gargle. Gargling causes the uvula and the vocal cords of the larynx to swell.
- Avoid hot liquids, as they cause the uvula to swell.
- Sip warm drinks to help the throat heal, and iced drinks to help control the pain. This may seem contradictory, but to get optimum relief of pain and swelling, you have to drink both.
- Use aspirin chewing gum (any flavor) to end pain.
- Take acetaminophen (Tylenol) or ibuprofen (Advil) for pain relief.
- Drink plenty of water to stay well hydrated.
- Try a warm-mist humidifier if your throat is sore from mouth breathing at night.
- Take papaya enzymes buccally, as described on page 207, to reduce inflammation and swelling in the throat and to reduce pain.
- Try antacids if GERD is a problem. Also, sleep on two

pillows or elevate the head of your bed to reduce the chance of irritation.

■ Do not eat after 8:00 P.M., and avoid caffeine.

■ Suck throat lozenges to relieve pain and keep your throat moist.

EAR PAIN

Otitis media means inflammation of the middle ear, resulting from a middle-ear infection. It can occur in one or both ears and many times is the result of inflamed and congested sinuses.

Causes of Ear Infection

In order to hear, we have an eardrum, which vibrates with sound. The three tiny bones located in the middle ear move back and forth in order to transmit the sound to the inner ear, where the nerves are. If the eardrum and the bones are to move properly, the middle-ear space has to have a pressure equal to that of the air outside the ear. But if you change altitude, the pressure outside changes, and the middle-ear pressure needs to be adjusted. This is done through the Eustachian tube (ET), which connects the middle ear to the nose and the outside. When you blow your nose too hard, this can close the ET, resulting in pain and pressure. In fact, any nasal congestion or sinus swelling can do this. A growth in the back of the nose can press on this opening, causing pain. Inhaled toxins can cause inflammation that leads to pain.

When your Eustachian tube is blocked, you may not be

aware that your hearing is impaired. In fact, many people think their ears are "plugged" when they actually have hearing loss. This occurs because the closure of the ET causes a vacuum to form in the middle ear, which prevents the normal vibration of the eardrum. If this closure persists, the body tries to fill this vacuum. The normal air-containing cells of the mastoid bone change to mucus-making cells, causing a condition called *serious otitis media*, or fluid filling the middle ear.

In a middle-ear infection, called *otitis media* (OM), the buildup of the pressurized pus in the middle ear causes earache, swelling, and redness. Since the eardrum cannot vibrate properly, you (or often your child) may have hearing problems. Sometimes the eardrum ruptures, and the pus drains out of the ear. But more commonly the pus and mucus stay in the middle ear. After the acute infection has passed, the effusion remains and becomes chronic, lasting for weeks, months, or even years. This condition makes you subject to frequent recurrences of the acute infection and may cause difficulty in hearing.

Diagnosing Ear Infections

Your doctor will start with a medical history and thorough physical examination. Then, using an instrument called an otoscope, the doctor will assess the condition of your ear. This will allow him or her to see whether you have fluid behind your eardrum or any redness indicating inflammation or infection. Other tests may be used if indicated, including an audiogram test, to check for hearing loss, and a tympanogram, to see whether the Eustachian tube and eardrum are working.

Treating Ear Infections

To relieve earache and unblock the ET:

- If your doctor prescribes antibiotics, take the full course.
- Use a nasal decongestant and guaifenesin (see chapter 10) to help mucus drain.
- Try papaya enzyme tablets—one tablet four times a day, dissolved in the mouth between the cheek and gum—to ease inflammation and thin mucus (see page 206 for more information).
- Drink at least six to eight cups of hot tea per day to thin mucus and reduce swelling.
- Be very gentle in trying to clear the ears because you can do more harm by forcing. The best method to use: hold the nose and try to *gently* force air out of the ear. Or put your tongue to the top of your mouth and swallow.
- Ask your doctor to prescribe analgesic eardrops if pain is a problem.
- Use analgesics such as ibuprofen or acetaminophen to reduce pain and inflammation.
- Use nasal irrigation to clear any nasal pus or infection.

If all other measures fail, ask your specialist whether an operation (myringotomy) may be helpful to promote drainage of fluid and reduce ear pain.

The Real Purpose of Earwax

Although you may not want to hear this, the human ear is very delicate. It is *not* designed for swimming, daily shampoos, hot tubs, or scuba diving. The human ear needs wax (cerumen) to protect against the ravages of soap and water. Unfortunately most of us are taught as children to scrub our ears with soap and water. Wrong! Or we've been told to use alcohol eardrops to dry up the moisture in the ear. Wrong again!

As annoying as it may feel, you *have* to have earwax. Once you pry and prod and clean the wax out of your ear canal, you have the equivalent of dishpan hands of the ear canal. Your ears will dry out and itch. Then, when you unknowingly scratch them in your sleep, infections start.

Doctor's Rx to Prevent Ear Itching

To prevent ear itching:

- Put five drops of baby oil in the ear canal before showering or washing your hair. This prevents any irritation caused by soap and water and helps keep the ear canal properly oiled.
- Take an over-the-counter antihistamine such as Benadryl at night to stop the itch and prevent you from scratching the ear in your sleep.

NO QUICK FIX, BUT THERE ARE ANSWERS!

Although there is no quick fix for the painful symptoms of sinus-related problems, you can find treatment success with a trial-and-error procedure. Work with your physician and try various medications and medical or complementary treatments to find the ones that will help. It will take some time while you sort through the options outlined in this book, but you will see greater benefits in the long run, as your painful sinus symptoms halt or even reverse.

Part Two

SEVEN EASY STEPS TO RELIEVING YOUR SINUSITIS

Chapter 4

STEP 1: MAKE THE DIAGNOSIS: TESTS YOU MAY NEED

You may be thinking, "After living with headaches and chronic congestion for years, there is no medication or treatment that can control my sinus problem." We're out to prove you wrong, and at the same time help you to halt or even reverse your sinus symptoms.

Unlike other books that tout a specific drug, food supplement, or nasal spray as the cure for sinusitis, we believe that there is no one set treatment. In fact, the most effective way to cure sinusitis, or at least to treat its symptoms, is to use a multidisciplinary approach. This involves making specific lifestyle changes, including changes in your diet and sleep habits, exercising daily, modifying your home and work environment to be allergen-free, keeping your sinuses irrigated and the harmful bacteria cleaned out, and using safe and effective medications. Yes, sometimes surgery is necessary for chronic sinus problems, but for most this is a last resort—after you've exhausted every other method.

The Sinus Cure's seven-step program will help you to finally put an end to the common and disruptive problem of sinusitis, but first it's important that you talk with your doctor and get an accurate diagnosis. When Ellen finally went to see an ear, nose, and throat (ENT) specialist, she had needlessly suffered from a congested nose and sore throat for more than two months. At age thirty-three, this young mother of two was exhausted all the time and felt achy all over, as if she had a low-grade fever.

After listening to Ellen's symptoms of chronic headache, purulent postnasal drip that choked her during sleep, and sharp pains in her ears that would come and go, the ENT did a physical examination and a few laboratory tests. He also did a CT (computed tomography) scan, which is a radiograph of the sinuses to see if infection, abnormalities, polyps, or tumors are present.

Ellen's doctor ruled out other more serious problems, and then diagnosed her with a chronic sinus infection. She started a three-week course of antibiotics, along with a seven-day pack of oral steroids to reduce inflammation and subsequent pain. Then she began to use other effective complementary treatments explained in this book. Even though she realized that there would be no instant end to the symptoms until the infection was cleared up, Ellen was relieved that finally she knew what was causing her headache and fatigue.

In today's high-tech medicine, we have become accustomed to using special testing, blood tests, or other expensive tests to arrive at a diagnosis. Yet with sinusitis most doctors begin the diagnosis by taking a thorough patient history.

EVALUATING YOUR SINUS PROBLEM

As you seek an accurate diagnosis of the cause and type of sinusitis, choose a doctor whom you can trust to take responsibility for your overall sinus health. This may be a general practitioner, an internist, an allergist, or an ENT specialist (otolaryngologist). If you have asthma or other lung problems, you may see a pulmonologist. Whomever you select, make sure the doctor is board-certified in this field. This means that the doctor has passed a standard exam given by the governing board in that speciality.

During the evaluation the doctor may perform the following:

- A complete physical examination, focusing on the nose, throat, ears, and neck
- A thorough check to see whether you have nasal polyps, swollen turbinates, or a deviated septum
- A check for signs of old fractures of the nose as well as enlargement of the tongue or elongation of the palate with swelling of the uvula
- An evaluation of nasal obstruction if the tip of the nose is depressed
- A check for open-roof syndrome in the nose because the nasal bones are separated and painful
- An evaluation of your ears and throat, looking for inflammation or signs of infection
- An evaluation of the head and neck, looking for swollen glands or abnormalities

Special tests such as a sinus CT scan may be ordered. This will allow your doctor to see in more detail the nature of nasal congestion or the anatomy of your sinuses. Of course, these additional tests will depend on your overall medical history, the physical examination, and what the doctor feels is necessary to better evaluate your problem. Keep in mind that your doctor should have a clear-cut therapeutic or diagnostic reason for all tests performed.

Your doctor will talk with you about your sinus symptoms, known triggers, your lifestyle, and past medical history. During this discussion, be open with your doctor about how you feel—when symptoms start, what makes them worsen, and what makes them end. It will enable the doctor to make a more accurate diagnosis, once the results of your physical examination, laboratory tests, or necessary X-rays are evaluated.

Your doctor will ask you to fill out a history sheet that includes the following:

- Past surgeries
- History of childhood allergies (pollen, mold, pet dander, dust, foods)
- History of eczema or asthma
- Gastrointestinal problems (acid indigestion, sour taste in mouth)
- Any drugs you are taking and the reason they are being taken
- Family history of allergy, diabetes, or cancer

THE EXAMINATION

In the examining room, your doctor will ask about your problems related to sinusitis, and much of the resulting diagnosis depends on your history. For example, if your problem is nasal congestion during the tree pollen season, that pretty much gives the diagnosis (allergy). If the pain in the sinus comes during the night and awakens you out of a deep sleep, it could be triggered by a migraine. Or if the pain between your eyes is relieved by decongestant tablets, that could indicate that the ethmoid sinus is involved.

Determining a Deviated Septum

The doctor will check the outside of your nose to determine whether it is crooked or deviated; then the nasal septum will be checked. Is part of the septum shoved against the side of the nasal cavity, blocking sinus drainage? Is it causing pain in your nose? Your doctor can identify any irregularities of the septum through examination and further testing. If the area where the septum impacts the turbinate is the cause of your pain, your doctor can anesthetize the area and correct the impaction.

Peering into Your Nasal Chambers

Using a nasal speculum and a lighted mirror, the doctor will peer far into your nasal chambers, looking for evidence of pus, swelling, inflammation, polyps, or even objects in your nose.

Checking the Turbinates

Your doctor will record the appearance of the turbinates (the shelves on the side of your nose, which can swell or shrink). Are they pale and spongy, indicating allergy? Are they very thin and crusted, indicating that the tissue is wasting away? The doctor will also note whether polyps are present.

Investigating the Throat

In the mouth and throat your doctor will check for diseases of the teeth, tonsils, uvula, and the back of the throat. He or she will make sure your tongue is free of disease and look for enlarged tonsils in back of your tongue called lingual tonsils, which could hinder breathing and affect your voice.

Your doctor will look for adenoid growth and assess the appearance of the Eustachian tube openings. Next the doctor will check for changes in the larynx, the vocal cords, and evidence of gastroesophageal reflux disease (GERD). There also may be large amounts of lymphoid tissue, which grows in response to the infectious drainage from the sinuses. There may be tissue in the back of the nose as well that blocks the sinus drainage.

Looking for Blockage in the Ears

Your doctor will examine your ears, looking for any signs of blockage of the middle ear. This may show up as the eardrum's being red and pulled inward by vacuum.

Checking the Sinuses

After spraying your nose with an anesthetic, the doctor will use a telescope with an angled lens to peer inside your nose and sinuses. The purpose of this is to check whether the following are wide open or blocked:

- The openings of the maxillary sinus called the maxilliary ostia (below the eyes and above the teeth)
- The openings of the frontal sinus (above the eyes)

■ The openings of the sphenoid sinus (way behind the eyes)

Evaluating Your Glands

The doctor will also check your neck for any swollen glands and evaluate the back and front muscles of the neck for any painful nodules. The doctor will see if your thyroid gland is enlarged or uneven as well, since this could play a key role in nasal and sinus problems. In certain conditions, such as hypothyroidism, you may be more prone to allergic reactions and sensitivity, which can lead to sinusitis. Sometimes allergy shots don't work, and your doctor will add a thyroid supplement to boost the effectiveness of the treatment.

Opening Wide . . .

The temporomandibular joint (TMJ) is also checked, along with the nose, throat, sinuses, and ears. The doctor will have you open your jaw to see whether it deviates on opening or whether there is cracking and popping at the joint. This will help determine whether TMJ syndrome is the source of your pain or discomfort.

Unfortunately, in the head, the pain may be caused in one area yet felt in another. For example, pain in the back of the neck is felt as frontal sinus pain. Tonsil pain is felt in your ear. You may have only a vague idea of your pains being a "headache," so your doctor will have to exhaust all the possibilities by checking various sites in the head and neck to find the true source of your pain.

TESTS YOU MAY NEED

We'd like to start off by saying trust your doctor to decide which set of tests is best in your case to ensure that no other medical problems are present. This can help you avoid extra testing that may add little to your diagnosis and only increase the number of tests and the expense. However, if you have a particular fear of one specific diagnosis, such as a brain tumor because of severe sinus headaches or cancer because of polyps, do tell your doctor. If you still do not feel comfortable with the diagnosis, talk to your doctor and then have more testing. Or get another opinion until you are confident that the problem has been diagnosed correctly. Then proper treatment can begin.

The following tests are commonly used to assess the degree of impairment and monitor the effectiveness of treatment.

Complete Blood Count (CBC)

Your doctor may ask for a complete blood count. This test measures the hemoglobin, red cells, white cells, and platelets, and can also find many of the common blood disorders, such as anemia, which can cause fatigue and tiredness.

The chemistries in your blood will also be checked and will include kidney and liver tests. The levels of cholesterol and other fat in the blood will be determined, as well as the level of calcium and other substances that can create problems that are similar to fibromyalgia but treated differently. Thyroid tests will be done at the same time as the blood tests to see whether the thyroid is working properly—or whether it is over- or underactive.

If you have serious lung disease with low oxygen levels in

the blood, the red blood cell count may be high. An elevated red cell count may lead the doctor to do further investigations of oxygen levels and lung function to help him or her decide how to improve your condition.

Sputum Examination

Special tests of mucus from secretions in the nose and lungs can be helpful in making a diagnosis and determining the best manner of treatment. Your doctor will look for certain cells in the mucus that indicate that allergic rhinitis may be the problem. Analyzing sputum coughed out of the lungs may also be helpful in diagnosing infections such as bacterial pneumonia or tuberculosis.

The Saccharin Test

Mucociliary clearance (MCC) is achieved by cilia, which help move out layers of mucus along the ciliated epithelium so you can stay well. In your upper respiratory tract, cilia propel the mucus and its trapped bacteria and particles to the nasopharynx, where it drops to the hypopharynx and is swallowed. In the lungs and windpipe, the cilia move the mucus blanket up to the larynx, where it is swallowed. Stomach acid then destroys the unwanted invaders.

When MCC is slowed down, mucus stagnates and bacteria begin to breed, setting the stage for infection and illness. In fact, decreased mucociliary flow is a regular precursor to sinusitis and lower respiratory infections. The saccharin test is used by many specialists to measure the mucociliary clearance. With this test a particle of saccharin or sodium saccharinate is placed in your nose behind the anterior edge of the turbinate. You are instructed to sit quietly and not sniff or snort.

Your doctor will ask you to swallow every thirty seconds and report any changes you notice. You will then be timed as to when the sweetness caused by the saccharin reaches the back of your tongue. The normal time is five to seven minutes. Nine to fifteen minutes is slow; sixteen to twenty-eight minutes is very slow.

Less than twenty-eight minutes shows that your condition is reversible, more than twenty-eight minutes is associated with permanent damage. A saccharin transit time of less than five minutes is seen when you are in the early stages of allergy.

Computed Tomographic Scan

A computed tomographic (CT or CAT) scan is a safe and effective test for producing detailed images of the nasal cavity and paranasal sinuses. It will show your doctor if the sinus openings are working or not and give a "reason" for symptoms you may be feeling. The CT study can show tumors, abnormal blood vessels, and infections, and can detect inflammation and obstruction in the sinuses. While the CT scan does involve a small amount of radiation, it is a quick and painless test.

Your doctor will perform a CT study when your sinus condition is under control. The reason for this is that inflammatory mucosa obscures the fine bony detail, which limits the usefulness of the resulting images. An MRI is not recommended because it is too sensitive, showing false positives that are really just mucus.

Saccharin Time Test Results

Saccharin Time (Minutes)	Speed	Clinical Indication
1–4	Fast	Acute allergy
5–7	Normal	Normal
10–18	Slow	Infection
19–25	Very slow	Chronic sinusitis
28+	Extremely slow	Irreversible; absence of MCC

Flexible Laryngoscopy

Flexible or rigid laryngoscopy is sometimes used to diagnose nasal and sinus disease or even tumors. It can also determine the response you may have to medical or surgical therapy. Your doctor will use a topical anesthesia, then pass a scope through your nose to view the nasopharynx and larynx. This procedure will help your doctor find problems in the epiglottis, vocal cords, and throat, along with any abnormal nodules, polyps, or tumors. If the back of the larynx is irritated, this usually means GERD (see pages 34–36).

Chest X-ray

Although a chest X-ray is not routinely required to diagnose sinus problems, if you also have symptoms of a cough that produces bloody sputum, your doctor may want this evaluation. Or if you are not responding to the treatment regime, this test may help to clarify the problem.

Chest X-rays usually show clear lungs for someone with asthma but may show various abnormalities if bronchiectasis, pneumonia, or other problems are present.

Spirometry Test

If you are having asthma symptoms (wheeze, chest tightness, cough) along with some sinus problems, your doctor may choose to do a spirometry test. This test measures how much air you can exhale and is the most accurate pulmonary function test used in confirming the presence of reversible airway obstruction.

When using the spirometer, you will be asked to breathe in and out of a hose attached to a mouthpiece. A small computer measures this amount of air on newer spirometers. The standard measurement is the *FEV-1*, or forced expiratory volume in one second. This is the amount of air exhaled in one second after taking a breath. This test can also monitor your response to medications and is recommended for adults and children older than age five.

Methacholine/Histamine Challenge Test

After you have taken the spirometry test, your doctor may say that you have a normal expiratory flow of air. However, please note that this does not exclude the possibility of asthma. Many of those with asthma have normal spirometry between attacks. So diagnosing asthma in these individuals requires some form of bronchial irritation to induce airway obstruction, and this is done by the methacholine/histamine test. This test is usually done in a pulmonary function laboratory. You will be asked to inhale a drug called methacholine in gradually increasing amounts. At each level of methacholine, spirometry will measure your breathing.

In a normal person, inhaling the methacholine has almost no effect. However, if you have hyperreactivity of the bronchial tubes, methacholine will cause bronchoconstriction and result in a decrease in expiratory flows. While the test is generally safe and easy to do, you may experience minor wheezing and chest tightness after inhaling this drug, which may require the use of a bronchodilator.

If the volume of air you can forcefully blow out in one second drops by 20 percent or more, and you also have episodes of shortness of breath, wheezing, or cough, this is certainly an indicator of asthma.

Allergy Tests

PAPER RADIOIMMUNOSORBENT TEST (PRIST)

The paper radioimmunosorbent test gives an accurate picture of the overall IgE (immunoglobulin E) level. IgE is an antibody that is bound to mast cells in the skin. A high level of this antibody can show if an allergy or an infection is present. Determining levels of the IgE antibody is also useful in assessing this response to treatment in certain cases of allergic disease. (Note: A normal IgE level, however, does not exclude the diagnosis of an allergic disease.)

QUANTITATIVE IMMUNOGLOBULIN DETERMINATION TEST

Quantitative immunoglobulin determination tests measure different immunoglobulin or antibody proteins in the blood.

This test provides clues about your immune system. If certain levels are low, it is easier for you to get a sinus infection.

A sample of blood is obtained for the measurement of levels of immunoglobulin. If the IgE levels are high, your doctor might consider an allergic cause for your symptoms, such as rhinitis or asthma. If the levels of other specific immunoglobulins are increased, then a certain infection may be suspected, such as pneumonia or a fungus. And decreased amounts of some immunoglobulins may signal problems with the body's immune system defenses against certain infections caused by bacteria or viruses.

RADIOALLERGOABSORBENT TEST (RAST)

The radioallergoabsorbent test is a blood test used in detecting IgE reactions to specific triggers. It is done in a test tube. While this test is no more accurate than skin tests (see the following subsection) at determining allergies, RAST may be considered for ultrasensitive persons for whom a skin test may pose a threat of a very severe allergic reaction. RAST is more expensive than skin tests, but it is not affected by the medications you may be taking.

SKIN TEST

Skin testing is suggested if there is a reasonable suspicion that a specific allergen or group of allergens is causing your chronic sinus symptoms. Skin tests involve injecting specific allergens under the skin to detect IgE-mediated responses. If an allergen reacts with the IgE antibody, then histamine may be released, and your skin will respond with redness and swelling.

There are several types of skin tests your physician may use, including prick, intradermal, and patch. The most common

Do-It-Yourself Allergy Test?

Although fancy medical tests are available for seasonal and food allergies, the best test may lie in your daily diary. For instance, if you start sneezing suddenly, instead of assuming you are allergic to the family dog, check the pollen calendar at www.pollen.com. This calendar gives the dates and amounts of various pollens in your area. If you have sneezing fits, nasal congestion, and hoarseness every time oak trees bloom, chances are great that you might be allergic to oak pollen. Or if you suspect a food allergy, write it down in your diary. When you eat the food again, see if you are symptomatic and write this down. If you do find you are allergic to fresh fruit or vegetables, usually you can eat them cooked or canned. The cooking process breaks down the protein so it's not the same.

is the prick method. Tiny amounts of allergens are dropped on your skin, usually on your back. A needle is then pricked through the skin into each extract. Within a period of less than fifteen minutes, a hive will appear at the specific site if you have IgE antibodies to the particular allergen.

Ear Exams

If sinusitis has resulted in a buildup of fluid in your ears and subsequent loss of hearing, your doctor may want to perform ear exams.

AUDIOGRAM—TO EVALUATE HEARING LOSS

An audiogram is a basic hearing test that checks on the pure tones you hear. Results are obtained by a trained audiologist in a special soundproof testing booth. A complete audiogram will test both the bone conduction (the ability to hear a sound when it is transmitted through bone) and the air conduction (the ability to hear a sound when it is transmitted through air). The louder the sounds have to be in order to be heard, the greater the degree of hearing loss.

The audiologist will compare the two types of conduction to see which part of your ear is responsible for any hearing loss. The results of audiograms are most often displayed in graph form.

TYMPANOGRAM—TO MONITOR EARDRUM MOVEMENT

This quick and easy test lets your doctor know how well the eardrum moves when a soft sound and air pressure are introduced into the ear canal. It is most helpful in diagnosing problems in the middle ear (like having fluid behind the eardrum).

The technician will put a special probe-like earplug in your ear. Then the specialized equipment will automatically record the data.

In a healthy ear, the middle ear is filled with air at a pressure equal to that of the surrounding atmosphere. However, if the middle ear is filled with fluid, the eardrum will not vibrate properly, resulting in a flat tympanogram. If the middle ear is filled with air yet this air is at a higher or lower pressure than the surrounding atmosphere, it will result in a shift of position of the tympanogram.

ELECTRONYSTAGMOGRAM (ENG)—TO TEST THE BALANCE FUNCTION OF THE INNER EAR

If you are having balance problems or dizziness along with your sinusitis, your doctor may order an electronystagmogram. This is not really a hearing test, but a test of the balance function of the inner ear. Using a small tube so your ear remains dry, the technician will run cool liquid followed by warm liquid through the ear canal. As the liquid changes temperature, the inner ear is stimulated, causing your eyes to make rapid reflex movements. The movements are documented and give the doctor information about your balance mechanisms.

A Test to Reveal Obstructive Sleep Apnea

If you snore and your doctor suspects a more serious problem of obstructive sleep apnea (OSA), you may be referred for a sleep study (polysomnography). Polysomnography is done at an accredited sleep disorder center. The sleep test is safe and painless, and will give your doctor necessary information about the oxygen drops associated with obstructive sleep apnea or other breathing problems. The sleep study may also tell if there are other diseases of sleep, such as thyroid disease, that account for your symptoms.

During the sleep study, the technician will monitor and record:

- Airflow at your nose and mouth
- Respiratory effort, signaled from monitors on the chest wall and abdomen
- Oxygen levels
- Leg movements

- Body position (supine, prone, side)
- Electrocardiogram (measurement of heart muscle activity)

If you are diagnosed with OSA, a treatment plan, including weight loss (for those who are overweight) and nightly use of CPAP (see chapter 2, pages 63–64), will be recommended, along with measures to treat the sinus disease.

Tests to Confirm GERD

If gastroesophageal reflux disease is thought to be the cause of your sinus symptoms, an esophageal manometry may be ordered. This test involves measuring the pressures inside the esophagus and stomach. A twenty-four-hour esophageal pH test may also be useful, as it verifies whether stomach acid refluxes into the esophagus. At times a special type of X-ray, called cine flouroscopy, may be necessary to see the esophagus and how it actually functions during swallowing.

ACCURATE DIAGNOSIS: THE FIRST STEP TOWARD EFFECTIVE TREATMENT

Getting back in control of your sinus symptoms starts with an accurate diagnosis. Once the type of sinus disease is properly identified, your doctor can prescribe a treatment regime that can halt, reverse, and even prevent your sinus problems.

Chapter 5

STEP 2:
TRY NASAL IRRIGATION

You've suffered from chronic sinusitis for as long as you can remember. Tired of taking strong antibiotics, you hear about nasal irrigation with saline solution (salt water) as an alternative to the standard round of prescribed medications.

You'd like to avoid taking drugs if possible. Yet you know that an infection needs aggressive treatment. A friend tells you about the yogic practice of nasal cleansing with saline solution, and you purchase a neti pot at your natural foods store. After irrigating the sinuses with the neti pot filled with mild saline solution, you are amazed at the instant relief you finally feel. All the bacteria-laden mucus is flushed out of your nose, and you can actually breathe clearly again.

You continue the nasal irrigation twice a day for three weeks. Each day you feel more improvement from the chronic sinus symptoms—less swelling, decreased headache pain, and no more cough. When you talk with your doctor, she explains that nasal irrigation improves ciliary function, and how the cilia—the basis of your body's natural defense against upper respiratory problems—will now work better to reduce stagnant mucus.

After three weeks, you are clear of infection. You now continue to use this natural therapy daily to prevent future infections and stay symptom-free.

Basically, nasal irrigation is just that—cleaning your sinuses out with a salt water (saline) solution. Although it may sound complicated, this easy-to-use and all-natural sinus cleansing method has many healing benefits, including the following:

- Removes bacteria, crusts, and pus from the sinus area
- Thins thick secretions so they can pass through the nasal passage
- Washes away pollutants and allergens
- Helps to reduce chest congestion that results from postnasal drip
- Reduces the bacteria breeding ground, leaving a better chance for natural healing without antibiotics

Beyond these benefits, nasal irrigation just feels good, as it establishes a more normal nasal environment through cleansing and added moisture. If you've ever had a stuffy, congested nose for days on end, you know how good it feels when you find relief and can breathe freely again.

Yet nasal irrigation is not a modern invention or New Age therapy. It actually goes back thousands of years to when Indian yogis used this method to cleanse their nasal passages. Although few studies have been done on alternative treatments for acute and chronic sinusitis, nasal irrigation is supported by many published clinical trials. In fact, the efficacy of using nasal irrigation to speed healing has been demonstrated in the orthopedic, surgical, and dental literature, too.

START WITH SALINE SOLUTION

Nasal irrigation depends on saline solution (salt water) to restore moisture to your sinuses and to reduce inflamed nasal membranes. A host of scientific studies show that if the saline irrigation is used regularly, it can help to keep mucus thin, decrease postnasal drip, and cleanse your nasal passages of bacteria.

Selecting the Right Solution

The type of saline solution you use is largely dependent on your particular sinus condition. For example, some scientific findings indicate that nasal tissues are healthier in isotonic solutions. *Isotonic* means that the solution contains the same concentration of salt as in your body. Most over-the-counter saline sprays are isotonic. Yet in some conditions of the nose, it is difficult to breathe because the nasal tissue is so swollen and edematous (retains fluid). A few researchers conclude that if you use a hypertonic solution (with a greater proportion of salt), some of the fluid may be pulled out of the swollen tissue, thus improving your breathing. It is thought that in some cases the fluid removed from the swollen tissues thins the mucus layer in which the nasal cilia move, helping to restore the cilia's function. This approach has been used to improve the function of chest cilia with promising results, and many people with severely swollen sinus passages have found great relief with hypertonic solutions. Still, if your nasal membranes are dry and crusted, thin and bleeding, a hypertonic solution may give adverse results, sometimes impairing cilia function.

So which solution do you choose?

Choose isotonic for dry sinuses. If your nose is dry and crusted, stick to isotonic saline. Baking soda is added to the saline solution to keep it from becoming too acidic and burning your nasal passages. A homemade isotonic saline wash can be prepared by mixing together the following:

1 pint (2 cups) warm water
1 teaspoon salt
½ teaspoon baking soda

(Some prefer to use pickling salt or kosher salt because of possible allergies to iodine, which these salts do not contain.) You can use regular tap water if it's clean, or any bottled water. It is not necessary to use distilled water.

Try hypertonic for nasal stuffiness. If your nose is stuffy, especially if it is stuffy at night before going to bed, try a hypertonic saline solution. The hypertonic solution has a greater salt concentration than the isotonic solution. Again, pickling salt or kosher salt is preferred by many sinus sufferers, and baking soda is added to keep it from burning your nasal passages. A homemade hypertonic saline solution can be prepared by mixing together the following:

1 pint (2 cups) warm water
2 teaspoons salt
1 teaspoon baking soda

When you try the hypertonic solution, go slowly. Gradually increase the amount of salt from 1 teaspoon per pint to 2 teaspoons per pint. Do not go above 3 teaspoons, as that can really burn.

Caution: Some sinus sufferers have difficulty with hypertonic

Pickled Fish and Your Voice

Did you know that the singer Enrico Caruso sucked pickled fish before giving a performance? The hypertonic solution diluted his mucus, making it easier to sing.

solutions, so be careful. Sometimes hypertonic saline solutions cause ciliostasis, a condition where the cilia stop functioning and may never recover. If the cilia are permanently damaged, the ability to fight infection is lost. If in doubt, ask your doctor before trying this to avoid irritating your nasal passage.

Using Saline Solutions

Now that you've prepared the right solution for your sinus condition, it's time to irrigate the nose. There are many different ways in which to use the saline solution. You can prepare the saline solution in a sterile plastic bottle, and then pour a small amount of the saline into your cupped hands. As you lean over the bathroom sink with your head down, inhale gently through one nostril, allowing the liquid to flow out of the nostril and your mouth. Do the same with the other nostril. Be sure to blow the nose very gently after each cleaning. You can also fill a large rubber bulb syringe with the saline solution. (If you have latex sensitivity, avoid using the rubber bulb syringe.) Or you can fill a commercial spray bottle with the saline solution and use this two or three times a day, especially when your nose feels either too dry or too stuffy. This is ideal after swimming in a heavily

Beware of Prepared Solutions
That Contain Additives

Many prepared saline solutions contain a host of additives and chemicals that serve as preservatives, antifungals, and antibacterials in order to give the product a long shelf life. Some of these additives include:

- Benzalkonium
- Thimerosal
- Monobasic sodium phosphate
- Dibasic sodium phosphate
- Phenylcarbinol
- Edetate disodium
- Povidone
- Disodium EDTA

The problem with additives in solutions you spray into your nose is that many people are highly reactive to the products, especially when they have a sinus condition or allergy. For example, in clinical trials in Sweden, researchers found definitive evidence that benzalkonium, found in several saline products, caused rebound rhinitis. When the benzalkonium was removed, the rhinitis was resolved. Other ENT specialists have experienced the same results. One doctor stated that 20 percent of adult patients cannot use the prepared over-the-counter saline solutions, and about 30 percent of children complained of burning and stinging with these products.

Many natural nasal sprays claim that the product kills bacteria. But, in fact, it is the benzalkonium preservative in the solution that kills the bacteria. When you remove this preservative, the product may have a different result.

The latest studies show that Ringer's solution, which is used intravenously in most hospitals, is the best solution for healthy cilia. A modified form of Ringer's solution is sold under the name Breathe-ease in the United States and SinuSal in the European Union. Neither of these products contains the additives listed above, but they do contain the electrolytes of Ringer's solution.

Alkalol, a nonprescription irrigating solution found at most pharmacies, is also healing for nasal irrigation. You can use this solution at about 2 to 3 tablespoons per pint of warm saline. Ask your doctor about other solutions that are available, and get a professional opinion on which solution—isotonic or hypertonic—is best for your sinus condition.

chlorinated pool or after exposure to industrial fumes or toxins. In all cases, throw away any solution that remains after a week, clean the bottle with very hot water, and prepare a fresh batch of saline solution.

Another form of nasal irrigation is to use saline solution with a neti pot—a ceramic container that looks like a genie's magic lamp. Neti pots can be purchased at many health food or natural food stores. Or you can check natural products Web sites on the Internet.

Fill the neti pot with the saline solution. Leaning over the sink, tilt your head to one side, and use the neti pot to pour the solution directly into one nostril. The solution will fill your nasal cavity and run out the other nostril and the back of your throat. Spit out this drainage, clear your throat, and gently blow your nose to clear the nasal passages.

Always keep in mind that your sinus condition may change from season to season. You may have to keep trying different variations of the saline solution each season until you get the perfect mixture that allows your sinuses to stay clear without infection. While most sinus sufferers prefer using isotonic solutions, hypertonic solutions work for some. Whichever solution you use, keeping the nose moist creates a healthier environment for almost every nasal or sinus problem.

HYDRO PULSE™ NASAL/SINUS IRRIGATOR

After doing years of research on sinusitis and related cilia dysfunction, Dr. Murray Grossan, a California-based ENT and the medical editor of this book, concluded that inhaling or sniffing saline solution at sixteen snorts per second is more healing than merely pouring saline solution in the nostrils. Based on his extensive published research and clinical trials, he invented the Hydro Pulse Nasal/Sinus Irrigator in 1976. With pulsatile irrigation, water is gently pumped into the nasal passages with a pulsating rhythm. Grossan believes this action stimulates the sweeping or waving motion of the nasal cilia.

Since Dr. Grossan's Hydro Pulse Nasal/Sinus Irrigator hit

the market, myriad subsequent scientific tests conclude that nasal cilia work better after irrigation, with improved breathing, fewer infections, and reduced chance of asthma. This simple attachment for the Hydro Pulse Nasal/Sinus Irrigator delivers saline at the right mixture, at the right pressure, and at the correct rate of pulsation to match the normal rate of the cilia. In test after test, pulsatile nasal irrigation has been found to be safe, even safer than blowing your nose.

As the saline goes through the sinuses and removes nasal crusts, pus, thick phlegm, and bacteria, the pulsation helps to heal the cilia, returning them to normal function. After you irrigate, your sinuses will contain the saline solution. This solution has displaced the mucus and bacteria that were in your sinuses. In about twenty minutes or so, the cilia will start to move on their own, resulting in the release of the saline. This shows that the saline went where you wanted it to go—into that sinus cavity.

Clinical trials involving thousands of men, women, and children of all ages have consistently shown that pulsatile nasal irrigation helps to increase blood flow to the nasal passages and restore function to damaged cilia. Because breathing is improved, there are fewer infections, and the chance of asthma is reduced. Clinical studies also report that regular nasal irrigation keeps patients from taking too many antibiotics, as stagnant mucus is regularly cleared out of the sinuses, reducing the chance of infection caused by bacteria. Obviously if there are fewer bacteria to contend with, you have a greater chance of clearing an infection without antibiotics, which is why many doctors use this for patient treatment.

For example, the journal *Patient Care* reported studies of patients with persistent or chronic sinusitis who used pulsatile nasal irrigation. The research concluded that this method is so effective in clearing the blocked passages that if done regularly, some of the patients needed no antibiotic treatment at all. In a study reported in *Transactions of the American Academy of Ophthalmology and Otolaryngology*, researchers found that patients with chronic sinusitis who used pulsatile nasal irrigation left doctors' offices with the bacterial load reduced, requiring fewer antibiotics and expressing much greater patient satisfaction. And still another study published in *Allergy: Principles and Practice* revealed that in patients with chronic rhinitis, the mucociliary transport is markedly increased after irrigating one or two times a day for two weeks with pulsatile irrigation.

For those who also suffer from asthma or bronchial problems, published studies indicate that irrigating the nose with saline solution may be helpful in restoring the cilia of the chest. In the journal *Otolaryngology*, research concluded that pulsatile irrigation improves both nasal ciliary function and chest condition. The chest is helped by the removal of the bacterial load from the nose and sinus. And sometimes asthma is caused or aggravated by pus in the nose, so using the irrigator to remove nasal sinus pus is beneficial.

In cases in which cilia are absent or nonfunctional (as in cystic fibrosis), the irrigation tends to act as a substitute for normal cilia. Even for healthy people, there are studies showing that regular use (three minutes a day) of a saline nasal irrigation may help you to resist colds. A groundbreaking report at the 50th Scientific Assembly of the American Academy of Family Physicians revealed that irrigation with saline solution prevents colds because it washes out a nasal substance called ICAM-1, to which the rhinovirus attaches to produce colds. Less ICAM-1 reduces the chance of a virus causing illness.

When Nasal Irrigation Is *Not* Recommended

It's important to note that while nasal irrigation with saline solution is a natural method of healing damaged cilia, it is not beneficial for everyone. Most sinus sufferers get excellent healing results from daily irrigation. Still, there are some people who should *not* use it. Do not use the nasal irrigation if :

- Your nose is filled with nasal polyps.
- The person using the device is younger than four years of age.
- You are having daily nosebleeds.
- You have just had nasal surgery (unless your doctor advises you to do so).

Always consult with your doctor before trying nasal irrigation or any alternative or holistic treatment.

It's important to note that not only does nasal irrigation clear out stagnant mucus, but its main function is to help restore cilia movement. Especially for those with thick postnasal secretions, nasal irrigation can stimulate healthy cilia and keep bacteria at bay. It is also helpful for postoperative cleansing following nasal or sinus surgery.

FREQUENTLY ASKED QUESTIONS ABOUT NASAL IRRIGATION

Q. *How often should nasal irrigation be used?*

A. Unless specifically recommended by your doctor, you should not irrigate more than twice each day. If your sinuses are healthy, you may not benefit from this at all. Talk to your doctor about your particular needs.

Q. *What if the saline gets in my throat during irrigation?*

A. It's important to have your head bent down into the sink so that the saline solution does not get into your throat. While there is no harm in this, this is not the intent. If the solution is going down your throat, you aren't leaning over the sink enough.

Q. *What if the saline stays in your sinuses?*

A. Nasal irrigation works when the solution goes into the sinuses and, after a period of time—about twenty minutes—the cilia start moving and the solution comes out of the sinuses. If your ears are affected, which is very rare, it means you are turning your head too much to the right or left. If you turn all the way to the left when you irrigate, then the opening to the right ear from the nose (the Eustachian tube) is at a point where the fluid can accumulate by force of gravity. Fluid can also get into the middle ear if it is wide open. Still, because you are irrigating with saline solution, it is easily absorbed. Or it will run out when your head is erect.

Q. *Should you ever add Betadine solution to the saline?*

A. Only if your doctor has recommended adding this.

Q. *Can I add my antibiotic to the saline solution?*

A. Again, only if your doctor recommends this.

Q. *What about agents that can be added to the saline solution that may help to cure fungal sinusitis?*

A. Unless your doctor specifically has suggested this, do not add anything to the saline solution. There are many Internet sites where people post remedies. Check with your doctor to make sure these are valid—and not hype.

Q. *What if my sinuses feel more swollen after irrigation? How do I get the saline to come out?*

A. There must be a lapse of about twenty minutes before all the saline will come out. This gives the cilia time to start functioning properly. If you are in a hurry, bend over and gently blow your nose. While leaning down, bend your head toward your right shoulder for one minute, then bend it toward your left shoulder for one minute. The liquid should properly drain out the nose.

Q. *Why can't you use nasal irrigation if you have nasal polyps?*

A. If your nose is blocked, it is highly traumatic to force fluid through it. A different approach is to treat nasal polyps. They usually respond to medications—a prescription of prednisone, the antibiotic amoxicillin, and steroid nasal sprays, as discussed on page 252.

Q. *Is it OK to use a vasoconstrictor nasal spray or inhaler to open the nose for irrigation?*

A Yes. The main thing is that you not use excessive force or pressure.

NASAL IRRIGATION AND ALLERGIES

For centuries, people have used the home remedy of rinsing the nasal passages with salt water to drain the sinuses. This is not simply an old wives' tale. Now scientists have found another benefit for this home remedy, concluding that good allergy management includes the use of irrigation for removal of offending particles and restoring normal ciliary flow.

In the *Journal of Allergy and Immunology*, researchers at the Department of Immunology of the Hospital Clínico San Carlos, Madrid, determined that daily nasal irrigation actually *prevents* the seasonal pollen allergy response of the body, which means avoiding suffering due to allergies.

Serum levels of immunoglobulin E (IgE) in response to pollen allergies increase in allergic patients during the pollen season. In the study, Drs. José and Javier Subiza tested a sample of twenty-five patients with allergies to pollen during the grass pollen season. During this season, the sample who performed pulsatile irrigation daily were checked for allergic response factors in the nose and in the blood and were also checked for inflammation in the nose. The patients who irrigated showed a significant reduction of IgE in the nose and in the blood, along with a reduction in inflammation. The observations show that the pollen and IgE had been washed out of the nose, actually preventing the allergic response.[1]

NASAL IRRIGATION AND SENSE OF SMELL

Studies show that regular nasal irrigation with saline solution improves olfaction or the sense of smell. Olfactory cells are

What Causes Loss of Smell?

Anosmia refers to complete loss of sense of smell. *Hyposmia* refers to reduced sense of smell. *Parosmia* refers to distorted sense of smell.

If your nose is blocked and you have anosmia, this may not be significant, as the nasal blockage may be preventing the smell particles from reaching the peripheral olfactory organ (organ of smell) located at the roof of the nose between the eyes. But if your nose is open and you have a sudden loss of smell, you should see a doctor as soon as possible. A common cause is a virus that promotes swelling of the nerves of the olfactory organ as they go through very narrow openings. Because this bone constrains swelling, the nerves may be cut off from nutrition and die. Immediate therapy with anti-inflammatory medication may save the sense of smell.

Other causes of loss of smell include aging, Alzheimer's disease, certain over-the-counter nasal sprays, chronic allergies, a cold virus, cystic fibrosis, drug side effect, endocrine disorders, excess smoking, exposure to formaldehyde, head trauma, heavy nose blowing, HIV infection, Huntington's disease, liver disease, Parkinson's disease, recreational drugs, rhinosinusitis, sarcoidosis, and work-related toxic substances.

found in a tiny piece of tissue high up in your nose. They connect directly to your brain and let you distinguish the fragrances of homemade bread, baby powder, and freshly brewed coffee—that is, when you can breathe through your nose!

Saline irrigation also improves the sense of taste. The gustatory cells are clustered in the taste buds of your throat and mouth. Because of these cells, you can discern if you are eating chocolate icing, sardines, or feta cheese—definitely importance differences!

If you've suffered a series of respiratory infections or have chronic, ongoing sinusitis, you know how your sense of smell and taste are affected. Each time you get an infection, these senses are the first to shut down. The sense of smell usually returns when the nose is cleared by nasal irrigation and the cilia return to good health.

NASAL IRRIGATION AND CHILDREN

What about children who suffer with endless colds, allergies, or resulting sinusitis? Nasal irrigation offers benefits for them as well. In a study published in *Clinical Pediatrics* on children five and older who had sinusitis, postnasal drip, or nasal blockage, those who used pulsatile nasal irrigation were able to remove the discharge, resulting in reduction of adenoid and tonsil hypertrophy (a noninfectious enlargement of these tissues that does not indicate a disease). Sinus irrigation also cleared the ear.

The most important thing you can teach your child in order to avoid future sinus problems is to blow the nose gently with both nasal passages open.

Proetz Sinus Irrigation

The Proetz method of sinus irrigation of the nose can effectively be done with children, even as young as eighteen months.

- Lay the child across the parent's lap. Extend the head back so that it is at about a 90-degree angle in relation to the body line.
- Drip several drops of ⅛ percent Neo-Synephrine saline into each nostril (available over the counter at most grocery or drug stores). Now fill both sides with saline.
- Aspirate using a bulb syringe with a nasal tip that seals the nose. The opposite nostril is occluded by the saline filling the nasal chamber.
- Continue filling the opposite side with saline and aspirating as the flow of the saline passes the sinus ostia until the return is clear. This acts like a water pump and suctions out pus and mucus.
- Proetz irrigation in this manner may be recommended by your doctor as a means of delivering antibiotics to your child's sinuses.

OTHER USES FOR IRRIGATION

Throat irrigation has been shown to significantly reduce the need for antibiotics, and to possibly obviate the need for tonsillectomy. It is also shown to prevent the spread of infection

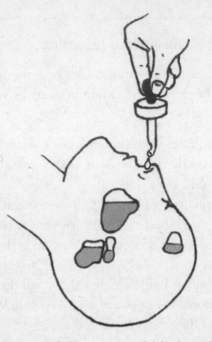

Demonstration of the Proetz method of nasal irrigation.

within the family. A condition called tonsillithiasis is characterized by white material sticking out of the crypts or holes in the
tonsils (see page 68). People worry needlessly about this because
it looks foul and produces bad breath. Irrigating the throat with
warm saline solution can help to remove this material.

In some cases, throat irrigation can safely replace gargling,
which may worsen some throat conditions. Numerous studies
have shown that gargling is ineffective and can cause laryngitis.

If your doctor has recommended surgery (see chapter 11),
nasal irrigation before sinus surgery has been shown to help reduce infection. Using irrigation after surgery may help to restore
ciliary function and reduce your symptoms.

Talk to your doctor and ask if nasal irrigation will help your sinus problem. Then try both the isotonic solution and the hypertonic solution to find which one helps to relieve your symptoms. Remember to continue the saline irrigation on days of heavy pollen or if you are having cold or allergy symptoms. This simple method of clearing the sinuses will help to flush thick mucus and bacteria and let you enjoy clear breathing again.

Chapter 6

STEP 3: CONSIDER COMPLEMENTARY TREATMENTS

After suffering with chronic sinustis and allergies most of my life, I had to find some answers. I found an allergist who believed in combining some alternative therapies with conventional medicine. With her guidance I eliminated foods I was allergic to and began to eat fish high in omega-3 fatty acids to help reduce the chronic nasal inflammation.

Then, using the combination of daily nasal irrigation, vitamins A, C, and E, and natural supplements to boost my immune power and improve the quality of my sleep, I regained energy and suffered fewer infections. I went from avoiding outdoor situations for fear of allergy attacks and sinusitis to going on power walks in a nearby park each afternoon before my kids got home from school.

—SHANNON, *age thirty-seven*

After undergoing two sinus surgeries, I still got frequent infections. I was sick of staying on prednisone and anti-biotics and was determined to get some sinus solutions that I could live with.

My ENT showed me some new studies on how drinking eight or more cups of water daily helps to keep the body hydrated, thinning mucus and making it easier to expel. She also gave me some natural papaya enzymes, which I take four times a day to keep inflammation down.

I now use saline nasal irrigation each day as well. Because my law career gets hectic at times, I've started to make time twice a day to use some relaxation therapies. I think that the combination of de-stressing and taking care of my body has enabled me to stay well and sleep sounder at night—another immune system booster. The result? No sinus infections in fourteen months.

—JACK, age forty-two

To combat my constant sinus headaches, I take the herb feverfew, which acts as an anti-inflammatory. Then I use hydrotherapy; the warm, moist heat opens up my sinuses so they drain. Now I have fewer sinus headaches as a result of increasing the drainage, and the headaches I do get are much less severe.

—SUE, age thirty-four

So where do you turn when you suffer from sinusitis—whether acute or chronic? If you're like most people, you run straight to the medicine cabinet and start popping the unfinished antibiotics you have from last year, thinking these "magic" drugs will be the cure. Yet after a few days of constant misery, you realize that just as it happened last year, these pills may ease the infection, but only if there *is* an infection. Antibiotics do not cure all the symptoms you may face with sinusitis.

But before you toss the unused portion of your antibiotics in the trash, it's important to realize that they are not all bad. Antibiotics *can* save your life, if used properly. An antibiotic works by stopping the growth of bacteria so your immune system can eliminate them or by directly killing the bacteria. Still, bacteria constantly develop resistance to the very drug that was designed to kill them. There may be only one bacterium in a large number of cells that is resistant to a drug; with the use of antibiotics every organism will be killed, except for that one. That lone survivor will continue to multiply and spread until it has replaced all the dead bacteria.

Comprehensive studies show that within six hours, a single bacterium can regenerate into a population of more than 1 million. According to the Centers for Disease Control and Prevention (CDC), in 1997 up to 25 percent of cases of streptococcus were not cured by penicillin. This figure has risen 11 percent in just four years. So when antibiotics are used too frequently, this can result in bacteria (germs) becoming immune to those antibiotics—all the more reason to consider complementary treatments if you suffer with sinusitis to manage the symptoms and keep infections at bay.

HOLISTIC TREATMENTS: A GROWING TREND

Many chronic sinus sufferers have discovered that a complementary approach to healing not only may give a boost to immune function, keeping infections at bay, but can also help to ease the accompanying symptoms of swollen nasal passages, headache, body aches, and fatigue.

We know that you, like most of today's consumers, are not waiting for your primary-care physician or even the latest government studies to outline a plan for the prevention of disease.

People want to take charge of their health and be involved in decision making regarding treatment methods, especially the 70 million baby boomers, who have always had a problem with authority (remember Woodstock?).

As forty-eight-year-old Linda said, "I'm tired of assembly-line medical care, where doctors spend an average of ten minutes at each visit. I want to learn some natural and effective ways to prevent, manage, or even cure my sinusitis." And Linda is not alone! According to a recent nationwide poll, more than four in ten adults in the United States (42 percent) now embrace alternative care therapies. The 1997 *Landmark Report on Public Perceptions of Alternative Care* reported that nearly half of adults in the United States (45 percent) say they would be willing to pay more each month in order to have access to alternative care. Of those Americans who use alternative care, almost three-quarters (74 percent) say they use it along with conventional medical care.

Within the realm of conventional medicine, there are some accepted alternative therapies—such as acupuncture, chiropractic, and nutritional foods—that many medical doctors will agree to use in conjunction with a traditional therapy. This does not mean that you should throw away your prescriptions. Instead, it means that *the two schools of healing—conventional medicine and complementary therapy—can work hand in hand to get you well sooner and keep you well.*

In fact, there is a growing trend at some of the nation's most prestigious teaching hospitals to blend the two schools of medicine. For example, Beth Israel Hospital in Boston recently set up a center for alternative medicine; Columbia University has done the same. Even the National Institutes of Health (NIH) has turned its head "cautiously" toward alternative treatments to sort out the truth from the hype. The NIH's Office of Alternative Medicine, headed by Dr. Wayne B. Jonas, is funding studies aimed at establishing or disproving the clinical basis for different types of alternative therapy. Yet while this marks a step in the right direction, the amount of money being spent to research unconventional treatments is still only about $14 million of the NIH's staggering $11 billion annual budget.

The Pros and the Cons

If you've never tried alternative therapies, it's important to keep in mind that the efficacy of most complementary treatments has hardly been proved. Talk with your doctor about the pros and cons of using each, and evaluate the benefit to your sinus condition and overall health. A good rule of thumb is to make sure the complementary treatment meets the following two criteria:

1. It makes you feel better.
2. It does not hurt you in any way.

Let's look at some of the most common forms of complementary treatment for sinusitis.

HYDROTHERAPY

Hydrotherapy is the use of water in all forms, from ice to steam, to promote healing. This complementary treatment works by stimulating your body's own healing force. Cold compresses reduce swelling by constricting blood vessels and helping to control minor internal bleeding. This is an excellent way to stop a nosebleed associated with sinusitis. Conversely, moist heating pads or warm, moist compresses on the sinus area can reduce the soreness and pain by increasing blood flow in and drainage out—an effective hands-on treatment for sinus headache pain or congestion.

So let's consider the commonly used forms of hydrotherapy for sinus ailments.

Moist Heat

Many sinus sufferers find excellent relief from clogged nasal passages and headache when they use twice-daily applications of moist heat. This is simple and inexpensive to do, yet the benefits are great. Not only will your sinus pain subside, but you will also help to increase drainage and blood flow to the sinus area.

The following are proved to be the most convenient and beneficial types of moist heat that may help sinus problems:

- Warm shower (also allows you to inhale steam, which can help to moisten and thin the mucus in your sinuses)
- Warm, moist towels placed on the frontal area (above the eyes), the ethmoid area (between the eyes), and the maxillary sinus area (below the eyes). Be sure to avoid direct contact on your eyes.
- Moist heating pad
- Hydrocollator packs (found at most drug stores)
- Hot water bottle with damp cloth

Use the application of moist heat twice every day, without fail. Start with ten to fifteen minutes each morning and evening. You may have to get up a few minutes earlier in the morning before work and allow time to do this before going to bed. The time spent is definitely worth the improvement you'll feel in reduced sinus pain and nasal congestion.

After three to four weeks, you may find that your chronic sinus inflammation or headache pain has lessened dramatically. Decrease the treatment to *one application* of moist heat to the sinus area each day. Then, as your level of pain, swelling, and congestion improves even more, use the moist heat only when you feel it is needed.

Hot/Cold Contrast Therapy

Alternate hot and cold applications on the sinus area. Using a damp cloth, alternate two minutes hot with one minute cold. Repeat four times, three times each day to reduce congestion and open the sinus area.

Water to Liquefy Thick Mucus

Drink tepid (room-temperature) water—and a lot of it. Just don't drink cold or iced water, as it stops the cilia from functioning normally.

Water keeps your respiratory system hydrated, which helps to liquefy thick mucus that builds up to cause infection in your sinus cavity. Some experts recommend drinking as much as twelve to fifteen glasses of fresh water daily, or even more. Keep a tall glass of water on your desk or pack a few extra bottles of water for work or recreation.

Other liquids can also be added, but don't depend on coffee, tea, or alcoholic beverages to make this goal. These liquids dehydrate the body of its water stores, leaving you needing even

How Much Water Do You Need?

To figure out the minimum amount of water you need each day, divide your weight in half. For every pound, drink an ounce of water you need each day. Add several more cups if your sinuses are problematic or if you exercise.

more water. In fact, those who are allergic to red wine, sulfites, yeast, or other components of alcohol face double trouble when they drink. Not only do they literally "dry up" from dehydration, but they also experience increased nasal allergies from ingestion.

Keep a few bottles of water in your car, by your desk at work, or where you sit to watch television to encourage drinking more.

Aromatic Steam

"When my sinuses are really congested, I keep a pot of water simmering on the stove," said Claire, age forty-seven. "As I'm cooking or working around the house in the evening, I stop by and inhale the steam for several minutes at a time. It keeps my sinuses open and draining and relieves any headache."

Some people with clogged nasal passages find great relief through breathing in steam. If you try this, be careful that you do not get too close to the steam, for you may get more than "clear breathing." Also, turn off the gas before you breathe in steam from heated water on a gas stove.

To gain optimum relief, try the following aromatic additions:

Natural Aromatic Relief

A natural product available at most health food stores is Tiger Balm. This ancient oriental remedy is filled with potent aromatic herbal extracts—menthol from peppermint, eugenol from cloves, cineole from cajeput (similar to tea tree), cinnamon, and camphor. Tiger Balm is rubbed into the sinus area, and some people claim it clears the sinuses instantly.

- Add two teaspoons chopped fresh ginger to the steaming water in a sink, warm-mist humidifier, or teakettle. First, let the ginger tea simmer for twenty minutes, then breathe in the steam for four to five minutes. Drape a towel over your head when breathing the steam to get maximum relief.
- Add one teaspoon of the over-the-counter ointment Vicks VapoRub to the steaming water, then breathe in the steam for several minutes or until you get relief.
- Add a few drops of oil of *Eucalyptus globulus,* peppermint, or menthol to the steaming water.

Definition of a Natural Dietary Supplement

According to the Food and Drug Administration (FDA), in order for an ingredient of a dietary supplement to be a "dietary ingredient," it must be one or any combination of the following substances:

- Vitamin
- Mineral
- Herb or other botanical
- Amino acid
- Dietary substance used to supplement the diet by increasing the total dietary intake (e.g., enzymes or tissues from organs or glands)
- Concentrate, metabolite, constituent, or extract

Herbal Therapy

If you have ever downed a cup of hot coffee and realized that it allowed you to breathe better, then you have tried herbal medicine. Herbal medicines include all parts of a plant—flowers, fruit, bark of trees, seeds, and vines—and are ingested in many forms. These natural compounds are used to treat ailments, such as ginger tea to fight off colds, echinacea and goldenseal to boost immune function and fight infection, or even coffee to open up swollen nasal passages.

Since ancient times, cultures have thrived on the use of plants and plant products for medicinal purposes. Traditional herbs are the backbone of Chinese medicine and are a common

Your Germ-Fighting Tool

The CDC and other public health experts agree that hand washing is the single most important means of preventing the spread of viral and bacterial infections, yet a study conducted in 2000 by the American Society for Microbiology revealed that about one-third of Americans using public restrooms in five major cities didn't wash their hands before leaving. Our hands come into daily contact with a multitude of contaminated surfaces, and when we touch our faces, germs can enter our bodies through our eyes, nose, and mouth. We can also transmit those germs by shaking hands or handling items that are then touched by others. Proper hand washing is sufficient to remove most of the bacteria from your hands, and here's how to do it:

- Run the water until it's warm.
- Wet your hands thoroughly.
- Apply enough plain soap to work up a good lather.
- Rub your hands together for 20 seconds, washing both sides of each hand, the spaces between each finger, and around rings, paying special attention to the areas around fingernails. (Whenever you have the time, it's a good idea to use a nailbrush, as bacteria tend to hide under your nails, and to keep your nails trimmed.)
- Rinse your hands thoroughly.
- Turn off the faucet without touching it if you can, because bacteria thrive on faucet handles.

(Depending on the type of faucet, you can use a paper towel, or maybe your elbow.)

■ Dry your hands thoroughly with a clean cloth towel, a paper towel, or an air dryer.

■ If possible, don't use your hands to open the bathroom door if in a public restroom. Either push it open with your shoulder or use a paper towel to turn the knob.

Also, wash your hands frequently throughout the day—before and after you eat, after using the bathroom, after gardening, before and after sex, and after handling any potential contaminants such as raw meat, unwashed vegetables, dirty diapers, or garbage.

element in Ayurvedic, homeopathic, naturopathic, and Native American medicine. According to the World Health Organization (WHO), about 4 billion people, or 80 percent of the earth's population, use herbal medicine to receive a desired benefit to the body. Although precise levels of use in the United States are unknown, in 1997 herbal products accounted for sales of more than $3.4 billion, the fastest-growing category in drugstores.

ESTABLISHING THE EFFECTIVENESS OF CAM

In response to the tremendous demand for natural therapies for healing, Congress formed the National Center for Complementary and Alternative Medicine (NCCAM) as part of the National Institutes of Health (NIH) to help appraise alternative medical treatments and establish their effectiveness. This organization is now creating safe guidelines to help people choose appropriate alternative and complementary therapies.

The fact is, the outlook for complementary and alternative medicine is remarkably optimistic, and we are gaining a better understanding of these nonstandard treatments and how they can increase health and prevent disease. Yet, in the midst of the appeal and mystery of natural therapies, don't close the door to conventional medicine, for this is where we all turn for the "big stuff." After all, who are you going to call when you have a bacterial infection, chronic illness, or need surgery? Your medical doctor should be at the top of your list for providing an accurate diagnosis and treatment for sinusitis.

Determining How Much Is Enough

Because each herb has a different property and purpose, you need to read the label or ask a practitioner for proper dosing. It is advisable to buy herbal supplements from a reliable company and make sure they have been standardized. This means the manufacturer has measured the amount of key ingredients in the batch. Don't forget that dosing is not exact with herbs, and the potency can vary. This is an important safeguard for you.

The whole herb consists of the entire plant processed into liquid or capsule form. Some herbs are in capsules made from a whole herb or an extract. These are easiest to store and are available at most grocery, drug, or natural food stores. Yet herbs can also come in liquids, either a tincture (made from the whole herb) or an extract (made from one or more parts of the herb). Extracts are usually diluted in a solution of water and alcohol and are more potent.

Herbs vary in price depending on where they are purchased,

how they are processed, and their strength. You may find that herbs that are calibrated or measured are also more expensive. Still, they may provide more of the healing element you are trying to ingest. If the herb is not calibrated, it may provide too little—or too much—of the active ingredient.

Exercising Caution

While herbs are natural substances, they can also be strong medicines. Most herbal products sold in the United States are not standardized, which means that determining the exact amounts of ingredients can be difficult or impossible. Some natural supplements and herbs are also highly toxic and can raise blood pressure, cause liver damage, and even lead to death—and because of the lack of regulation by the government, most consumers would not know this until they ingested the product. For example, as Socrates realized, the poisonous plant hemlock is very natural but also very deadly! There are *nine herbs* that the FDA currently lists as *considered unsafe*: chaparral, comfrey, germander, jin bu huan, lobelia, magnolia, ma huang, stephania, and yohimbe.

Also, if you are facing upcoming sinus surgery, the American Society of Anesthesiologists (ASA) advises that you avoid the following herbs in the two to three weeks preceding elective surgery, due to complications that may occur: feverfew, garlic, ginger, ginkgo biloba, ginseng, kava-kava, and St.-John's-wort.

Now check out the list of herbs, in the next subsection, that are used holistically for the treatment of sinusitis and related respiratory problems. If you decide to take herbal supplements, play it safe: talk to your doctor, a pharmacist, or a certified nutritionist about side effects. *Note:* Herbal therapies are *not* recom-

---

The USP Mark of Reliability

Always select reliable brands for your dietary supplements. Make sure these brands are stamped with a USP mark (United States Pharmacopoeia, an independent nonprofit organization that sets public quality standards for prescriptions, over-the-counter medications, dietary supplements, and other products). This mark on the product's label signifies that the USP has tested and verified the ingredients, product, and manufacturing process.

---

mended for pregnant women, children, the elderly, or those with compromised immune systems.

HERBS COMMONLY USED TO REDUCE INFLAMMATION

By classification, natural supplements contain substances such as vitamins, herbs, minerals, and amino acids. A number of these supplements inhibit the body's inflammatory compounds such as leukotrienes, substances released from the membranes of mast cells during the IgE-mediated reactions that cause the uncomfortable inflammation, bronchoconstriction, and excessive secretion of mucus.

Because chronic sinusitis is an inflammatory disease, the following herbs have been found helpful in reducing inflammation and decreasing symptoms:

- *Boswellia.* This herb, commonly found in Ayurvedic medicine, has been used for centuries as an alternative to aspirin. While there are limited findings on this herb for rhinosinusitis, a few studies suggest that boswellic acids may possess anti-inflammatory activity at least as potent as common over-the-counter medications such as ibuprofen and aspirin.

  It's thought that boswellia inhibits pro-inflammatory mediators in the body, such as leukotrienes. In patients with sinusitis, boswellia may reduce overall body aches, sinus headache, and ear pain, and also help to decrease sinus inflammation. *Caution:* May cause slight gastrointestinal effects.

- *Nettle.* This herb has been used for years in Germany as a safe natural therapy. Nettle contains a variety of natural chemicals that may help to lower inflammation and pain. These chemicals also help slow down the actions of many enzymes that trigger inflammation, such as cyclooxygenase and lipooxygenase. *Caution:* Excessive amounts of nettle may cause stomach irritation, constipation, or burning skin. If you are allergic to pollen, avoid nettle.

- *Turmeric.* Turmeric contains a strong anti-inflammatory compound, curcumin. Responsible for the yellow color of Indian curry and American mustard, turmeric is a member of the ginger family and a native of southern Asia (probably India). Whole turmeric is more powerful than isolated curcumin.

  It is thought that turmeric works similarly to COX-2 inhibitors to decrease inflammation by lowering histamine levels and possibly by increasing production of natural cortisone by the adrenal glands. *Caution:* May cause gastrointestinal problems. If you are taking anticoagulant medications, drugs that suppress the immune system, or nonsteroidal pain relievers (such as ibuprofen), you should avoid turmeric.

■ *White willow.* This plant provides another natural approach to treatment for chronic sinus headaches. The bark of the white willow tree is a source of salicin and other salicylates, compounds that are similar in structure to aspirin (acetyl salicylic acid).

Salicylic acid blocks inflammation, the body's response to injury and illness. In a study published in the *British Journal of Rheumatology*, researchers compared the effectiveness of willow bark (in the form of the product Assalix) with a COX-2 inhibitor. Both groups reported a decrease in pain. Researchers concluded that there was no significant difference in effectiveness between the two treatments at the doses chosen, but treatment with white willow bark (Assalix) was about 40 percent less expensive. *Caution:* White willow bark has the same potential as aspirin to cause gastrointestinal upset and have a blood-thinning effect. Do not take white willow bark along with aspirin or other nonsteroidal anti-inflammatory drugs.

Herbs Commonly Used for Sinus and Nasal Problems

■ *Anise.* Use seeds, dried herb, or capsules as an expectorant for getting rid of phlegm. Anise has an antiviral effect in large doses. It has a pleasant taste when used in tea form.

- *Astragalus*. Use dried herb, capsules, or tinctures to stimulate the immune system with an antiviral effect. It boosts white blood cell activity, and some proponents believe it helps to bolster resistance to disease. *Caution*. Astragalus may cause loose stools or abdominal bloating.

- *Black cohosh*. Use dried root, capsules, or tincture to help treat fatigue and sore throat or as an expectorant. *Caution:* Because of its estrogenic effects, black cohosh should be avoided by pregnant women. Do not use it if you have heart disease.

- *Borage*. Use seeds, leaves, flowers, whole plants, or supplements to soothe mucous membranes of the throat, sinuses, and mouth. Borage also stimulates the adrenal glands, helps to restore energy, and is used to treat bronchitis and digestive system upsets. Borage is safe if used according to package directions.

- *Butterbur*. Findings published in the *British Medical Journal* (January 2002) indicated that butterbur works as well as a conventional treatment for hay fever. In this study, researchers from Switzerland compared butterbur to the antihistamine Zyrtec (cetirizine) in a double-blind trial. Butterbur has also been found useful for prevention of migraines. *Caution:* Use PA-free butterbur extracts only. Pyrrolizidine alkaloids (PAs) are toxic to the liver.

- *Coffee*. Use dried whole beans, ground beans, liquid, or instant forms as a decongestant and to help ease congestion due to sinusitis, colds, and flu. As a bronchodilator, it helps to prevent asthma attacks. A preliminary test has found that heterocyclic amines, a new class of protective elements, are found in both caffeinated and decaffeinated coffee. These elements may work like antioxidants to protect against cancer, heart disease, and diseases associated with aging. *Caution:* Keep in mind that coffee is addictive and can cause withdrawal symptoms, which can last several days. It causes insomnia, increases anxiety, and can irritate the stomach lining.

■ *Echinacea.* Use supplements, tincture, liquid, powder, or foods (cough drops) to stimulate the immune system and ward off colds, sore throat, or flu. Echinacea stimulates the production of interferon, a natural body substance important for the body's defense against disease. It has been found to increase levels of properdin, a natural compound that helps to destroy viruses, fungi, bacteria, and other disease-causing microbes. Be sure to follow package directions for the correct dosage. It may take about one week before you notice a difference. Take echinacea intermittently, as the effectiveness wears off after eight weeks of continuous use. *Caution:* Echinacea may trigger allergic reactions in some people. It is not recommended for those with autoimmune diseases such as lupus, and the majority of medical studies conclude that echinacea works best to treat illness, not to prevent it.

Herbal practitioners recommend that if you purchase echinacea at a health food store, you perform a mouth test before buying. Ask the clerk to let you taste the echinacea product to see if it produces a

---

Remember the Letter G for Cold or Flu Relief

Goldenseal, garlic, ginseng, and ginger are all powerful virus fighters. Use these in hot teas or as supplements for optimal relief.

"buzz" in the mouth. These experts claim that lack of reaction indicates a weakness in potency.

- *Elderberry*. Use capsules to prevent respiratory tract infection. Elderberry contains the compound sambucol, which may help to ease flu symptoms.
- *Eucalyptus*. Use dried bark, seeds, leaves, or aromatic oils to help clear sinus congestion, bronchitis, asthma, croup, and chest congestion. The aromatic oils from eucalyptus halt bacterial growth.
- *Feverfew*. Use dried plant, tablets, or capsules to inhibit inflammation and fever and to slow the blood vessel reaction to vasodilators like prostaglandins. It acts similarly to aspirin. Use feverfew to treat chronic headaches. Take it daily to help with pain and inflammation. Or make feverfew tea by steeping one teaspoon of dried plant in two cups of water for fifteen minutes. *Caution:* If you have a clotting disorder, consult your physician before taking feverfew.
- *Garlic*. Use dried cloves, powder, oil, supplements, or capsules for antimicrobial, antiviral, antibacterial, and immunostimulating properties. Garlic gives some relief from cold symptoms and upper respiratory prob-

lems by stimulating the mucus-producing vagus nerve reflexes. It releases a powerful antibiotic called allicin. Garlic supplements may vary in potency, so follow package instructions. Some like garlic best if swallowed with applesauce or yogurt. If you do not chew the garlic, you will not "wear" it on your breath. *Caution:* Large amounts of garlic can reduce blood-clotting time and can be dangerous for those taking anticoagulants.

■ *Ginger.* Use dried root, tea, extract, tablets, or capsules to stimulate mucus-producing vagus nerve reflexes. Ginger contains nearly a dozen antiviral compounds, including several called sesquiterpenes, which help to fight cold viruses. It has an antioxidant and anti-inflammatory effect and stimulates the production of interferon. Add half a teaspoon of cayenne pepper to ginger tea to boost the effect.

■ *Ginseng.* Use tea, powder, capsules, tablets, or extract to help stimulate special enzymes that promote the elimination of toxic foreign substances. May help to increase the immune response by stimulating the number of antibodies in the body. *Caution:* Ginseng can cause headaches, insomnia, anxiety, breast soreness, or skin rash. More serious side effects include asthma attacks, heart palpitations, increased blood pressure, or uterine bleeding.

■ *Goldenseal.* Use dried root, capsules, or tincture to soothe inflammation of the respiratory, digestive, and genitourinary tracts caused by allergy or infection and to enhance mucous membrane function. Goldenseal contains at least two active constituents—berberine and hydrastine—that can help fight sinus infection. Gargling with goldenseal soothes a sore throat. *Caution:* Pregnant women, people with hypoglycemia, children, and the elderly are advised not to take goldenseal.

- *Horehound*. Use dried herb, tincture, and concentrated lozenges to relieve bronchial complaints related to sinus or postnasal drip.
- *Horseradish*. Use grated, fresh, or prepared to help clear nasal congestion and promote drainage. Add a teaspoon or two of horseradish to your sandwich at lunchtime. Try wasabi, a hotter Japanese horseradish, for an extra kick. *Caution:* Sometimes spicy foods can worsen sinus drainage, especially if you have allergies. The spices stimulate the flow of histamine.
- *Hyssop*. Use dried or as a tincture to relieve coughs, congestion, hoarseness, and mucus buildup. It is valued for loosening phlegm in the lungs and throat. Follow package directions to make hyssop tea. Add a teaspoon of sage to the tea to increase decongestant properties. *Caution:* May cause diarrhea or upset stomach.
- *Licorice*. Use root, syrup, lozenges, or cough drops to soothe mucous membranes. Licorice also helps to thin mucus and alleviate sore throats, coughs, and asthma. *Caution:* Licorice can cause stomach distress, diarrhea, and fluid retention. Large amounts of licorice can lead to a sudden increase in blood pressure. Use licorice root with potassium if high blood pressure is a concern.
- *Mullein*. Use dried leaves, stems, flowers, and oil as an expectorant and antitussive to relieve respiratory

problems such as asthma, bronchitis, and sinus congestion. Relieves dry, bronchial coughs. Use oil of mullein to treat ear pain. *Caution:* You may have mild stomach upset or diarrhea with mullein. Do not take mullein if you are pregnant or nursing, or have a history of cancer.

- *Myrrh.* Use resin, tincture, oil, or powder for an antibacterial action that relieves sinusitis, respiratory congestion, asthma, coughs, and colds. Gargle with myrrh tea for irritated mouth or throat. *Caution:* Large amounts of myrrh may cause laxative action, sweating, vomiting, kidney problems, and rapid heart rate.

- *Peppermint.* Use dried peppermint leaves, crushed herb, oil, tea, or extract to relieve nasal, sinus, and chest congestion. It stops cough by increasing saliva and freshens the breath. *Caution:* Peppermint is not recommended for children younger than age five or for those with acidic stomachs.

- *Pycnogenol.* Use supplements, dried root, or tincture to help alleviate symptoms of hay fever and many allergies. This antioxidant is said to contain a special blend of water-soluble bioflavonoids to boost immune function and reduce the formation of histamine and inflammation. *Caution:* In some chronic conditions, such as lupus, Pycnogenol has been found to worsen the illness.

- *Sage.* Use as tincture, dried, and capsules for an antioxidant and antimicrobial to kill bacteria and fungi, even those resistant to penicillin. Sage dries up phlegm and relieves coughs and throat irritations. Use as a tea, mixed with other herbs to cut the harsh flavor. *Caution:*

Sage can cause convulsions in high doses. Pregnant women should not use it at all.

- *Saw palmetto.* Use as capsules, tincture, and fresh or dried berries to relieve nasal congestion, asthma, bronchitis, and cough. Use according to package directions.
- *Slippery elm.* Use powder, dried root, supplements, or lozenges to relieve sore throat and soothe mucous membranes. *Caution:* Some people are allergic to slippery elm.
- *Spirulina.* Use whole plant, tonic, or supplements to aid in allergy control and boost the immune system.
- *Thyme.* Use oil or the entire plant to remove mucus from head, lungs, and respiratory passages. It helps to fight infections. Thyme is found in toothpastes, gargles, and mouthwash products such as Listerine.

HERBS FOR FLU SYMPTOMS

While there is no instant cure for the flu, a few herbs may help take the misery out of your symptoms. Elderberry is an ingredient in patent medicines in Israel, where one study showed that it decreases the duration of flu symptoms and prevents the flu virus from invading respiratory tract cells. Use echinacea with goldenseal for a powerful antiviral action. Or mix ginger tea using 1 teaspoon fresh grated ginger root in 1 cup boiling water. Steep for 10 minutes, then strain.

HERBAL COUGH SYRUP

To calm a cough associated with sinusitis or cold virus, try the following herbal recipe:

½ teaspoon cayenne pepper
½ teaspoon fresh grated ginger root
2 tablespoons honey
2 tablespoons apple cider vinegar
4 tablespoons water

Mix, and take by the teaspoon. Store in refrigerator.

SLEEPY TIME HERBS

When sinusitis robs you of sleep, you awaken feeling frazzled and anxious. The following herbs can sufficiently calm you down without causing you to feel drugged. Be sure to talk with your doctor before taking any natural dietary supplement as some may interact with other medications or cause an allergic reaction.

- Chamomile (*Matricaria recutita*). Chamomile depresses the central nervous system and also boosts immune power. Chamomile increases relaxation, promotes quality sleep, and can be used to relieve anxiety.

  Use chamomile as dried herb, supplements, and herbal tea. When making chamomile tea, steep the dried herb or tea bag for 5 to 10 minutes in hot water, and drink this three or four times a day. *Caution:* If you have ragweed allergies, chamomile may exacerbate your symptoms.

■ Passionflower (*Passiflora incarnata*). This herb is useful as a sedative, antispasmodic, and mild pain reliever. Passion flower may help to ease insomnia, stress, and anxiety. A study reported in the July 2001 issue of the *Journal of Clinical Pharmacy and Therapeutics* concluded that passion flower may decrease pain, which may help those with painful sinus headaches.[1]

Passionflower is available as tincture, fruit, dried or fresh leaves, or capsules. Follow package directions for dried herb in capsules. *Caution:* Avoid combining passionflower with prescription sedatives, and do not take if pregnant or nursing.

■ Valerian (*Valeriana officinalis*). Valerian has a sedative effect and may be useful in treating insomnia, particularly in helping to reduce the amount of time that it takes to fall asleep. Valerian is regarded as a mild tranquilizer and has been deemed safe by the German Commission E for treating sleep disorders brought on by nervous conditions. Unlike prescription or OTC sleep and anxiety medication, valerian is not habit-forming, nor does it produce a hangover-like side effect.

Valerian is available as capsules, tincture, and dried flowers. To ease sleep and combat insomnia, the usual dosage of valerian extract in tablet form is 300 to 900 milligrams taken an hour before bedtime. For stress and anxiety, the recommended dosage is 50 to 100 milligrams taken two to three times each day. *Caution:* Avoid taking valerian with alcohol, certain antihistamines, muscle relaxants, psychotropic drugs, sedatives, barbiturates, or narcotics.

Add Good Bacteria with Antibiotic Therapy

If you or a family member is taking antibiotics for a sinus infection, talk to your doctor about acidophilus capsules or powder to replenish the body with good bacteria. These bacteria are often called probiotics and serve to maintain the health of the intestinal tract by producing acids and other compounds that inhibit the growth of disease-causing bacteria. You can purchase acidophilus at any natural foods store.

HOMEOPATHY

Fight pollen allergy with pollen? Sounds a bit odd, but homeopathy is a naturopathic form of medicine that is based on the principle of "like cures like symptoms." This means that remedies that would cause a potential problem in large doses will actually encourage the body to heal more rapidly if given in small doses. Vaccines work on this principle, as they introduce small doses of an illness-causing agent to cure or prevent disease. Allergy shots work in the same manner.

Herbal preparations come from plants but are used in a "potent" concentration. Homeopathic remedies are made from plant, animal, or mineral substances, but only the most dilute substances are used so that only the smallest, most effective traces remain. Unlike herbal treatments, homeopathic remedies are regulated by the Food and Drug Administration (FDA). While there are several scientific theories on why homeopathy works, many believe that the principle of "like cures like" operates on a subtle yet powerful electromagnetic level, gently acting to strengthen the body's healing and immune response. A homeopathic solution must be "activated"—a process called succussion—to make sure that the original substance is diluted.

Homeopathic medicines may have benefit for:

- Allergic rhinitis
- Hay fever
- Migraine or sinus headaches
- Allergic asthma

There are studies showing homeopathy's benefits for asthma. Also, patients who received extremely dilute preparations of their primary allergen reported significant improvements within one week. Whether it will help your sinus symptoms is another story, but still, some sufferers find it beneficial, especially if they also have asthma or allergies.

Lack of convincing scientific proof is one of the great problems with homeopathy's acceptance by conventional medical doctors. Critics believe that because the medications are so diluted, the only benefit received is a placebo effect. Nonetheless, a survey of 107 clinical trials published in the *British Medical Journal* showed that 80 percent were in favor of homeopathy. Other studies in British journals provided evidence that homeopathic remedies are beneficial in treating allergies, asthma, migraine, flu, and hay fever. One landmark review published in *The Lancet* said that homeopathy was shown to be nearly two and a half times more effective than placebos in the treatment of such problems as arthritis, allergies, varicose veins, and gastrointestinal pain.

If you want to try homeopathy for sinus problems (see page 161), consult with a medical doctor (M.D.) or an osteopathic doctor (D.O.) who uses homeopathic treatments, and check in with this doctor as needed. Ask where he or she studied homeopathy and whether a certification exam was passed. M.D.s and D.O.s are certified by the American Board of Homeotherapeutics ("D.Ht." follows the person's name). Nurses, chiropractic doctors, and acupuncturists can receive their Certification in Classical Homeopathy (C.C.H.). Your insurance company is more likely to cover homeopathic treatment if the person rendering the service is a health professional (M.D. or D.O.).

Dosing is individualized, and two to three days of treatment is usually sufficient for most conditions. The doses generally come in the form of liquid drops, syrups, tiny sugar pills, or ointments that are diluted to various strengths or potencies. If you do not find relief within twenty-four hours, try another remedy.

Caution: Because of the possibility of allergic reactions, check with your primary-care physician before taking any unknown substance or supplement that promises great cures.

CHIROPRACTIC

Chiropractic is still another alternative method of treating sinusitis, particularly when congestion and sinus headache are concerns. According to chiropractic doctors, your nervous system controls all functions in your body. Every cell in your body is supplied with nervous impulses, and messages must travel from your brain down your spinal cord, then out to nerves to the particular parts of the body, then back to the spinal cord, and back up the spinal cord to the brain. The theory is that abnor-

Common Homeopathic Remedies
for Sinus-related Problems

Remedy	Ailment
Allium cepa	Allergy, cold
Ambrosia	Itchy, watery eyes; congestion
Apis	Sore throat, upper respiratory infection
Arsenicum	Asthma symptoms
Arundo	Watery or itchy eyes, runny nose
Belladonna	Sinus pain, swelling, and congestion
Bryonia	Headache
Chamomilla	Earache
Euphrasia	Allergy
Gelsemium	Headache
Hepar sulfur	Sinus infection
Histaminum	Itching, swelling, and overall allergy response
Kali bichromicum	Stringy postnasal drip, sinus pain
Mercurius	Sinus pain
Natrum mur	Hay fever
Sabadilla	Sneezing, watery eyes
Solidago	Runny nose
Spigella	Sinus pain
Wyethia	Itching throat, difficulty swallowing

mal positions of the spinal bones may interfere with these messages and often are the underlying cause of many health problems, including sinus drainage, sinus congestion, and sinus headaches.

Doctors of chiropractic correct the abnormal positions of the spinal bones with what is called an adjustment or spinal manipulation. The doctor's hands or a specially designed instrument delivers a brief and accurate thrust. This adjustment involves the use of a specific force in a precise direction applied to a joint that is fixated, locked up, or not moving properly. Adjustments help return the bones to a more normal position or motion, relieving pain and ill health.

For those suffering sinus-related ear problems, some believe that chiropractic may relieve the problem of blockage in the middle ear by using subtle adjustments. When used with conventional medicine, chiropractic maneuvers may help to increase normal drainage, which reduces infection and sinus headache pain.

ACUPUNCTURE

Acupuncture is the insertion of very fine needles on your body's surface in order to influence a physiological response. A specialist places very thin, sterilized stainless steel needles into your skin at different points on the body. Using heat, pressure, friction, suction, or electromagnetic impulses to stimulate these points, the practitioner may also turn the needles.

According to advocates, natural energy, or *chi* (pronounced "chee"), travels along fourteen pathways (or meridians) in the body to keep your body nourished. These meridians are connected to specific organs and bodily functions. When *chi* is blocked or thrown off balance, illness or symptoms result— in your case, sinusitis. The acupuncturist stimulates the points along these meridian lines, using the needles to remove the energy block and restore balance and flow of energy along the pathway.

With the inserting and twisting of the tiny-gauge needles at different points on your body, it is believed that acupuncture causes the body to release endorphins. Endorphins are the body's natural "calming" hormones, which may add to the feeling of relaxation. A hormone that fights inflammation is also produced in the body and may be triggered during acupuncture, which could explain why those with chronic neck or sinus headache pain have found relief. Some studies even suggest that acupuncture may trigger the release of certain neural hormones, including serotonin, which add to the feelings of calmness.

Moxibustion is used in conjunction with acupuncture. This is done by applying heat to the specific acupuncture points on the body. Many have found moxibustion helpful for bronchitis or asthma.

In 1996, acupuncture needles were recognized as "medical devices," meaning that your insurance company is more likely to cover this complementary treatment. This may vary depending on state regulations, licensing, and medical supervision, so check it out ahead of time. The National Institutes of Health (NIH) consensus panel on acupuncture has recommended that it be covered by Medicare.

ACUPRESSURE AND REFLEXOLOGY

Acupressure is a well-known ancient Chinese medical therapy that was discovered before acupuncture, using the same points. This noninvasive form of massage therapy is performed with the fingers or a hard, ball-shaped instrument. It works by stimulating your body's main "trigger points" to release energy or unblock *chi* with the hands instead of needles. Zone therapy, or reflexology, is also based on unlocking the body's energy blocks. With reflexology the soles of your feet and ankle joints are stimulated by hand.

Acupressure and reflexology allow you to apply pressure to specific points on your sinuses, head, and neck with the goal of alleviating pain and increasing drainage. While some find that using acupressure relieves their sinus headache, caution is advised. If you press a nerve that is on a bone or held in place by a bony canal, you can cut off the circulation to that nerve. The nerve could become irritated or even die, leaving you with additional pain and a lifetime of suffering.

MASSAGE

If you suffer with sinus headaches or facial pain due to congestion, you know how pressure applied at different parts of the face and neck can bring relief. Massage and bodywork techniques may help your body's natural ability to counteract pain by stimulating the brain to produce endorphins.

Massaging your sore sinuses brings a fresh blood supply to the area and soothing relief. Try pressing your thumbs firmly on both sides of your nose and hold for ten to twenty seconds.

Just be careful of pressing too hard on your face or neck, as you may damage delicate nerves, resulting in more pain than you originally had. Ask your doctor to recommend a certified massage therapist to see if this alternative therapy may keep you pain-free.

MOVEMENT THERAPY

As discussed in chapter 3, there are many causes of headache. Sometimes what you may think is a sinus headache is actually referred pain from the back of your neck. Whatever the cause, certain neck exercises may help.

Before and after you exercise, stand in the shower with the back of your neck to the shower nozzle. Let the flow of warm water run on your neck for five to ten minutes as it helps to loosen the tension. As the water is massaging painful neck muscles, gently turn your head to the left. Then turn your head to the right very slowly. Slowly lean your head into your shoulder, side to side. Lean your neck forward, then backward. Always be gentle and let the water provide a warm massage.

NASAL STRIPS FOR
NIGHTTIME CONGESTION

If sinus swelling and drainage keep you from sleeping well at night, nasal strips may help to alleviate this problem. The Food and Drug Administration has approved Breathe Right nasal strips to help relieve congestion and nasal stuffiness. These strips of tape are placed over the bridge of the nose, then a plastic strip springs back, helping to gently open your nasal passages and reduce air-flow resistance. This drug-free measure to improve breathing is also said to help reduce snoring to some extent in some people who wear these strips. Breathe Right nasal strips come in three sizes and are available in most pharmacies and grocery stores.

Another method of opening the valve in the nose to en-courage nighttime breathing is to use 3M surgical tape, one-quarter inch wide. Gently apply one end of the tape to the tip of your nose, lift, and fasten the other end of the tape to the top of your nose. The relief you feel may be well worth the effort!

THE POWER OF BELIEF

Whatever complementary therapy you choose, it's important to know that the power of belief in healing is massive. It was once estimated that about one-third of all healing occurred simply because the patient believed the treatment would work. This is called the *placebo effect*. Some researchers theorize that as much as two-thirds of all healing occurs because of the pa-tient's positive beliefs. Placebos have proved effective in reliev-ing the very real symptoms of colds, headaches, seasickness, angina, anxiety, and postoperative pain. So why not sinus prob-lems, too?

Having a sense of control over your health is also vital to wellness. That's why it's important to take charge of your sinus health by learning all you can about this common ailment, along with the many ways to treat it.

Ask questions about treatments that some may consider alternative or nontraditional. See what effect the treatment may have. Also ask about dangerous side effects. Then, along with your doctor-prescribed medications, use the alternative treatments in a complementary manner—in a way that enhances both health and well-being.

Chapter 7

STEP 4: CLEAN UP THE AIR AROUND YOU

"I can't wait until summer, when I can finally breathe again." Lynn's chronic sinus problems had plagued her since childhood, causing constant headaches and thick postnasal drip that kept her throat irritated and made her cough all night. These symptoms were exacerbated during springtime, and Lynn stayed exhausted from lack of sleep and chronic sinus headache pain.

"My sinus congestion coincides with the spring pollen. When the pollen count rises, I know to call my doctor for medicine. Then, as the oak blossoms appear, the sinus swelling and drainage escalate. Even on medication, I end up blowing my nose and coughing up thick mucus for weeks until the pollen season ends."

Coughing, sneezing, wheezing, choking, pressure, and pain—sinus sufferers put up with a lot of misery. Unfortunately you can't control some environmental triggers, such as the change of seasons, a cold front, or the pollen count. Still, there are other factors that play a key role in sinus health, including where you live, your work environment, the air you breathe, and what you do for a hobby or recreation.

Environmental triggers vary from person to person and can even change for the same person. But generally molds, pollen, dust, animal dander, internal and external pollutants, and chemical toxins are key triggers that greatly affect sinus health. No matter what is wreaking havoc on your sinuses, there are proven methods to control or even eliminate these offenders.

EVALUATING YOUR AIR QUALITY

Let's dig in and figure out what is causing you so much pain, congestion, fatigue, and overall distress. First, you have to check out the air you breathe each day. No matter how new or clean your home or office, minuscule particles—dust mites, pollens, molds, and animal dander—are entrapped in tightly insulated and poorly ventilated areas. These pollutants permeate the air around you and may trigger your clogged, drippy sinuses. If allergy is a problem, pollutants will give you a double whammy of sneezing, wheezing, and sinus pain.

Although you might have hoped that the newly built, tightly insulated home in which you live would be a surefire way to keep sinus problems away, that may not be the case. One comprehensive study found an allergen level to be 200 percent higher in a tightly insulated home as opposed to a home that is not as well insulated.

"Hey, but my house is *clean*. I dust each week." Wrong again. Even though you may have removed the visible dust from the furniture, there are tiny organisms called dust mites that live all over your home. In fact, dust mites are the most common cause of perennial allergic rhinitis (see page 24)—which frequently goes hand in hand with your sinus problems. Dust mite allergy usually produces symptoms similar to pollen allergy and also can produce symptoms of asthma.

Consider the facts:

- Dust mites are tiny bugs related to spiders that measure about one-hundredth of an inch in length. These minuscule creatures feast primarily on a diet of skin scales.
- Dust mite waste causes chronic allergic symptoms in more than 20 million Americans; an estimated 500 million people around the world are allergic to dust mites.
- Fifty to 80 percent of all asthma cases are triggered by dust.

Now that you know that the cleanest air can still harbor "mighty" sinus triggers, add to your "sinus pollution" a host of chemicals you innocently use to wash clothes, clean bathtubs, and put that gloss on wood furniture. While popular brands of these chemicals are sold in colorful cans at grocery stores, most can cause a host of respiratory problems, including inflamed and clogged sinuses, resulting in sinus headache and congestion. If you have ever sniffed bleach while washing clothes or inhaled pine cleaner in an enclosed area, you already know how chemicals can trigger problems with your airways.

The World Health Organization estimates that 20 to 30 percent of office workers around the globe suffer from some form of sick building syndrome, with more than 30 percent of new or refurbished offices putting them at risk. Because of well-built homes, there is a good chance the air you breathe at night is sick, too. Sick air equals sick sinuses.

Other environmental exposures that can add to your sinus misery include:

- Ragweeds, pollens, and grasses
- Cooking ingredients such as flour or spices
- Aerosols
- Chemical fumes
- Cigarette smoke
- Cold air
- Fresh paint
- Humid air
- Mold and mildew
- Perfume and scented products
- Pet dander
- Pollen
- Tobacco smoke and wood smoke
- Weather fronts
- Wind

Taking Charge of the Air You Breathe

Once you've assessed your home and work environment, use the following strategies to clear the air. It's important to control any sinus triggers that you can.

Strategy 1: Win the War against Dust Mites

Although dust is a key player as the cause of many sinus and allergic symptoms, studies show that *decreasing your exposure can also help to decrease your symptoms*. Remember that rather than a single substance, house dust is a mixture of different materials—

and all have the potential to trigger allergic reactions. The dust in your home may contain:

- Fibers from fabrics
- Feathers or cotton lint
- Dog or cat dander
- Bacteria, mold, and fungus spores (especially in damp areas)
- Food particles
- Bits of plants and insects
- Cat urine

If you've ever seen sunlight streaming through an open window, you have seen the biggest culprit—those tiny flecks in the sunlight are microscopic dead dust mites and their waste products. One gram of dust may contain as many as 250,000 dust mite feces, and it is this waste that makes your sinuses inflamed.

What can you do to win the war? The following preventive measures can help you eliminate as much of this waste as possible and reap the benefit of healthier sinuses.

START IN THE BEDROOM
The highest levels of dust mite allergen in your home are found in the soft surfaces of the bed. Because you spend so much time in close contact with your bed and pillows, it makes sense to start in the bedroom to clear the air. Here's what to do:

- Measure the level of house dust mite infestation with a dust mite detection kit, such as AcloTest. This is available in most allergy supply catalogs, or you can ask your pharmacist to order it.

- Most dust mites live in your mattress, so encase the mattress in a special allergen-impermeable casing. These casings are now available as tightly woven fabrics rather than the plastic of the past.
- Encase your pillow in a plastic zip-on cover to stop this allergen in your bedding. These can be purchased at any allergy supply store. Tape over the zipper to seal out dust leaks. If you do not want to use a pillow cover, wash your pillow in hot water (130°F) every two weeks to remove dust mite buildup. Also wash your sheets, pillowcases, and covers in hot water each week.
- Use blankets made from fabrics such as Vellux, acrylic, or cotton thermal. The latest covers are soft and silky in texture. Avoid all down-stuffed pillows or comforters, and never use a feather pillow if you have allergies of any type.
- Remove all carpeting and heavy drapes from the bedroom. Replace carpet with tile, wood, or linoleum, and damp-mop the area every few days to keep mites to a minimum. Tile floors do not provide the soft nesting areas that carpets do.
- Use central air-conditioning during warm and hot months. This will filter the air, taking out more than 99 percent of all the pollen and allergen-producing material it contains. It will also help to prevent the high heat and humidity that stimulate dust mite and mold growth.
- Ask your AC service contractor to install electrostatic air filters to help stop dust mites, pollen, and mold spores from blowing out of the room vents. Electrosta-

tic air filters remove particles (down to 0.01 micron in size) by static electricity and create an electrostatic charge as air passes through the special filter material, which causes it to attract and hold contaminant particles. Also ask your AC service contractor to inspect the air ducts in your bedroom and your entire home, and consider having these professionally cleaned.

■ Dust at least once a week, or more often if possible. Wear a dust mask when you clean, use nonporous vacuum cleaner bags, and get a vacuum with a high-efficiency particulate-arresting (HEPA) filter to help eliminate dust. HEPA filters are efficient in filtering out almost 100 percent of airborne allergens and danders.

■ Use several layers of cheesecloth as a filter over incoming air vents. These will help to trap dust, dirt, or lint coming through the ductwork. Change the cheesecloth filters every few weeks.

■ If possible, keep clothing in another room to lessen dust in the bedroom, and always keep closet doors shut.

■ Launder your clothes frequently. Dust mites thrive in clothing where perspiration provides a moist environment. While a cold water wash will get rid of some dust mites, only hot water will kill the mites.

■ Avoid moth flakes and room deodorizers, as they may trigger an allergy or a sinus reaction.

■ Purchase a HEPA room-sized air filter for your bedroom. These air cleaners are effective in removing irritating pollens, dust mite allergens, mold spores, pet hair and dander, tobacco smoke, bacteria, and house dust.

MAKE CHANGES IN YOUR HOME AND WORK SPACE

But don't concentrate only on the bedroom area. Other parts of your home need your focus, too! You may want to consider doing the following:

- Replace dusty carpets with linoleum or hardwood floors, and moldy curtains with shades or easy-wipe shutters.
- Use a solution of 3 percent tannic acid to neutralize the allergen in dust mite droppings. Acarosan (benzyl benzoate) can be purchased at an allergy supply store or through allergy mail-order catalogs. This powder is sprinkled onto carpets and vacuumed after it has dried. Acarosan eliminates house dust mites and their larvae, while separating and binding house dust mite excrement particles together for easy removal by vacuuming.
- Keep your house cool (less than 70°F) and dry (less than 50 percent relative humidity). Both measures help decrease the abundance of dust mites, as well as cockroaches and fungal problems.
- Purchase a humidity gauge to let you know when your home is too humid (more than 50 percent), as mites grow best at 70 to 80 percent humidity and cannot live in less than 50 percent humidity. Optimally, humidity in your home should be below 40 percent to prevent dust mite infestation.
- Purchase a dehumidifier to keep the indoor humidity below 40 percent, but be sure to clean this regularly. Fans might help, too, but keep the exhaust blowing toward the outside.
- Maximize the airflow inside your home, along with re-

ducing the dust and mold, by leaving doors open between the rooms.

■ Avoid using humidifiers and vaporizers, as they can increase the dust mite and mold growth. If you use these, be sure to empty and clean them daily.

Strategy 2: Stop Mold and Mildew

Jake's sinus problems began after a two-week camping trip in Colorado last summer. "I've always suffered with seasonal allergies. Still, I never had a full-blown asthma attack caused by sinus inflammation until I tried camping.

"I inherited a camper from my uncle and couldn't wait to take my family on a two-week camping trip. The first night we set up camp, I volunteered to check out the campsite. Within minutes of walking around in the woods that humid night, I was congested and coughing from the drainage in my throat. I couldn't sleep all night because I couldn't breathe. By morning I was wheezing from the chronic cough and drove into the nearby town to see a doctor.

"The doctor diagnosed me with sinobronchial syndrome, which is bronchitis triggered by a sinus condition. She put me on antibiotics and a decongestant. Then she handed me some sample asthma inhalers to control the wheezing and warned me to go home, sell the camper, and stay in a motel next time we travel to avoid humidity, pollen, and mold."

More and more people are taking advantage of outdoor recreation with hiking, camping, biking, rappelling, white-water rafting, or canoeing. Yet as Jake discovered, these outdoor activities may give you more than a good time—if the air is humid and filled with mold and mildew.

Mildew is caused by molds, which are parasitic, microscopic fungi without stems, roots, or leaves. Mold spores appear outside after spring and reach their peak from midsummer to October. In the South and on the West Coast, mold spores can be found year round. And molds are present almost anywhere. Outside, they can be found in soil, rotting wood, vegetation (such as wet leaves or mulch), vinyl furniture, cushions, patios, and boat canvas. Inside, molds are found in bathrooms, bedrooms, refrigerators, garages, attics, garbage containers, carpets, damp wallpaper, rotting wood floors, and upholstery.

Even the most well-built home or office building can be a haven for moisture, mold, and mildew—and therefore a cause of your unending sinus symptoms. A study published in the *European Respiratory Journal* concluded that exposure to moisture was significantly associated with sinusitis, acute bronchitis, nocturnal cough, nocturnal dyspnea (breathing difficulty), and sore throat. Exposure to mold or mildew was also strongly associated with the common cold, cough without phlegm, nocturnal cough, sore throat, rhinitis, fatigue, and difficulties in concentration.

To prevent molds in your home and work space, you have to find ways to dry out the dampness. This means providing good ventilation, light, dryness, and cleanliness for your home and office. Consider the following antimold measures as you work to eliminate sinus triggers:

- Keep your kitchen and bathroom surfaces dry. Use diluted bleach, if necessary, to remove any mildew in musty areas. If bleach is irritating to your sinuses, wear a mask or let someone else do the cleaning.
- Fix any leaky pipes or cracks and crevices to avoid water leakage in the home or office.

- Reduce indoor humidity to less than 40 percent to keep mold down.
- Purchase an ultraviolet light that will eliminate mold spores when it is on. These are used in hospitals to kill bacteria and viruses, but mold spores are also sensitive to this wavelength.
- Try silica gel (available under different trade names) to stop mold growth by absorbing moisture from the air. This is a mixture of activated alumina and calcium chloride. Set the container in a closet, basement, or damp area to absorb excess moisture.
- Change your home or office air filter at least every other month, or consider changing to a HEPA air filter to improve air quality.
- If your home is damp, use a dehumidifier to help reduce the humidity and mold levels. Check your basement for hidden mold and mildew.

Strategy 3: Watch Out for Pollen

Allergic rhinitis, which affects more than 15 percent of all Americans, often leads to sinusitis and is primarily caused by pollens. These microscopic powdery granules from flowering plants are the mechanisms for fertilization of trees, grasses, and weeds. Every plant has a specific period of pollination. Although weather changes can determine the pollen count in the air, the pollinating season stays constant.

Allergy and asthma sufferers must cautiously watch those dry, hot, or windy days when pollen is heavily distributed. In fact, because pollen travels for great distances, many different trees, grasses, and weeds can cause problems—not just the ones in your yard.

Some researchers have found an association between pollen allergies and food allergies. There is evidence that a family of proteins called profilins, which are present in many plant species, are capable of acting as panallergens. Profilin sensitization from birch tree pollen and other pollens has been shown to cross-react with sensitization to many fresh fruits and vegetables.

During times of heavy pollen, it is important to follow a few rules to avoid sinus congestion or infection:

- Stay inside and keep your windows closed, especially during heavy pollen times. Peak pollen and mold time is at 5:00 A.M., then again at 5:00 P.M.
- Shower, wash hair, and change clothing after being outdoors.
- Use air-conditioning, which cleans, cools, and dries the air.
- Keep car windows closed to avoid pollen during travel.
- Purchase a portable HEPA air filter for your bedroom. Air filters clean the air that passes through the filtration system. Many people who use HEPA filters report feeling better with reduced sinus or allergy symptoms. Filters need to be changed regularly in freestanding units.
- Consider allergy shots to reduce hypersensitivity (see pages 257–259).
- Hire someone to take care of your lawn during peak pollen season.

- Be aware of the pollen count, which is usually shown in weather reports on TV or on the Internet.
- Always premedicate and take reliever medications with you in case of breathing emergencies, no matter what the pollen count.

Strategy 4: Avoid All Smoke

If there is one step to take in controlling your sinusitis, this is it: *avoid smoke*. Not only does this mean don't smoke cigarettes, for that is a given for overall health and disease prevention, but it means avoid *all* smoke: secondhand smoke (the smoke from a burning cigarette and the smoke exhaled by a cigarette smoker), smoke from your barbecue grill, smoke from your oven when food has boiled over, or smoke from an outdoor or indoor wood fire.

Smoking greatly raises the risk of all types of health problems and is the major cause of emphysema, chronic bronchitis, and lung cancer. Not only is the smoker exposed to the health hazards of this destructive habit, but passive, or secondhand, smoke exposes innocent bystanders to poisons such as benzene, formaldehyde, and carbon monoxide. Sidestream, or secondhand, smoke, the smoke you inhale from someone who is smoking, has even higher concentrations of some harmful poisons than the mainstream smoke inhaled by the smoker.

Smoking increases the risk of sinusitis and other respiratory problems, but it is *one* important environmental risk factor that you can control. While you cannot control the fact that springtime blossoms cause allergy and sinusitis, *you can avoid smoking*.

IF YOU SMOKE: *QUIT*. Make a commitment *today* to stop. Cigarettes contain nicotine, a stimulant and an addicting

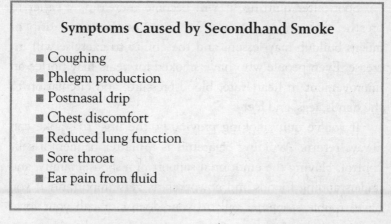

Symptoms Caused by Secondhand Smoke

- Coughing
- Phlegm production
- Postnasal drip
- Chest discomfort
- Reduced lung function
- Sore throat
- Ear pain from fluid

drug. After you stop smoking, the chances are great that you will feel irritability, nervousness, and headaches for one to two weeks, especially if you have been a heavy smoker. The newer nonprescription nicotine patches that are worn on the skin, nicotine gum, or other prescription medications can help you through the difficult period of withdrawal, helping to make the physical problem less troublesome.

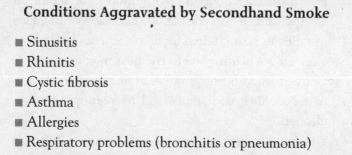

Conditions Aggravated by Secondhand Smoke

- Sinusitis
- Rhinitis
- Cystic fibrosis
- Asthma
- Allergies
- Respiratory problems (bronchitis or pneumonia)
- Ear infections

Soon after quitting, it will become increasingly easier to breathe through your nose. The constant postnasal drip or mucus buildup may lessen, and the ability to exercise will increase. Even people who have smoked for years may notice an improvement in heart rate, blood pressure, and circulation to the hands, legs, and feet.

If you've quit smoking previously, the urge to smoke can always return. Avoiding cigarettes is a matter of mental self-control. Having the emotional support of a spouse, family, and understanding friends and coworkers is very important. If you have trouble stopping, talk to your doctor or call your local chapter of the American Lung Association or the American Cancer Society. There may be a branch of Smokers Anonymous at your local hospital, which can offer great support in kicking this deadly habit.

Many types of smoke can irritate sensitive sinus passages. So take the following precautionary measures to breathe free and avoid sinus infection:

■ Avoid being around smoke from an indoor fireplace, wood-burning stove or heater, or outdoor barbecue grill. If you cook on a gas stove, consider purchasing an electric unit. If you cannot do this, have ceiling fans installed in your kitchen for better air circulation.
■ Convert gas heating to electric heat in your home.
■ Convert wood-burning stoves or fireplaces to electric to reduce dust and smoke and to keep the kitchen cleaner.
■ Designate a smoking area in your home, such as the back porch.

- Make sure your workstation is away from smokers.
- Leave rooms where people are smoking cigarettes, and ask for meetings to be held in a well-ventilated room.
- Always choose the "no smoking" section of restaurants and public places.
- Purchase a HEPA filter to help absorb smoke and chemical gases.
- Ask coworkers to leave the room when they smoke.

Strategy 5: Stay Away from Pets

Most pets can cause allergies, especially cats and dogs. If you also have sinus trouble, pets present a double whammy, making you cough, sneeze, itch, wheeze, and drain. Cats usually produce more severe allergic reactions than dogs do, but both species affect approximately 15 percent of the population and 20 to 30 percent of those with asthma. Some recent studies have even suggested that male cats are more likely to make you sneeze. Fur and skin tests showed that females produced one-third fewer allergy-causing proteins (allergens) than males. The production of cat allergen is thought to be triggered by the predominantly male hormone testosterone.

You may be allergic to a protein found in the saliva, dander, or urine of the animal. When the animal grooms, this allergen is carried through the air on invisible particles, then lands on the lining of your eyes and nose. It may be inhaled directly into the lungs. Pet allergies can also affect the skin, causing hives and itching. The animal's hair or fur can collect dust, pollen, mold, or other allergens and bring them into the home.

When Smokers Quit

Within twenty minutes of smoking that last cigarette, the body begins a series of changes that continues for years:

In twenty minutes
- Blood pressure drops to normal.
- Pulse rate drops to normal.
- Body temperature of hands and feet increases to normal.

In eight hours
- Carbon monoxide level in blood drops to normal.
- Oxygen level in blood increases to normal.

In twenty-four hours
- Chances of heart attack decrease.

In forty-eight hours
- Nerve endings start regrowing.
- Ability to smell and taste is enhanced.

In two weeks to three months
- Circulation improves.
- Walking becomes easier.
- Lung function increases up to 30 percent.

In one to nine months
- Coughing, sinus congestion, fatigue, and shortness of breath decrease.
- Cilia regrow in lungs, increasing ability to handle mucus, clean the lungs, and reduce infection.
- Body's overall energy increases.

In one year
- Excess risk of coronary heart disease is half that of a smoker.
- Skin is less wrinkled and dry.

In five years
- Lung cancer death rate for average former smoker (one pack a day) decreases by almost half.
- Stroke risk is reduced to that of a nonsmoker five to fifteen years after quitting.
- Risk of cancer in the mouth, throat, and esophagus decreases to half that of a smoker.

In ten years
- Lung cancer death rate is similar to that of nonsmokers.
- Precancerous cells are replaced.
- Risk of cancer to mouth, throat, esophagus, bladder, kidney, and pancreas decreases.

In fifteen years
- Risk of coronary heart disease is that of a nonsmoker.

Source: American Cancer Society and National Centers for Disease Control and Prevention.

Bird droppings are another source of dust, fungi, mold, and bacteria. The droppings of other caged pets, such as hamsters or gerbils, also breed these allergens.

Try the following preventive measures if you have a pet:

- Keep your pet outside your home. If you find this difficult, at least keep the animal out of your bedroom. Even if you do remove the pet, it can take weeks to months before all the pet allergen is gone.
- Keep all animals clean, and wash them weekly in lukewarm water without soap. Studies show that this may reduce the amount of dander and dried saliva deposited on furniture and elsewhere.
- Let nonallergic family members or friends bathe the animal and clean the bedding, litter box, or cage.
- As a last resort, consider finding a new home for that beloved pet if your symptoms are chronic.

Strategy 6: Steer Clear of Inhaled Fumes and Chemicals

Many sinus sufferers are greatly affected by fumes, inhaled chemicals, or other types of irritants. Even your makeup, shampoo or conditioner, or deodorant could affect your sinuses because of added perfumes.

The following measures can help you avoid problems arising from chemical intake:

- Make sure your home or office has good ventilation.
- Purchase new equipment, as improved equipment design can reduce the production of vapors, mists, and splashes. Enclosing of equipment can keep fumes from polluting the air.
- Replace or re-cover furniture, as some fabrics give off chemical smells, especially formaldehyde, which can irritate eyes, nose, and breathing passages.

Avoiding Air Pollution

Studies have found that exposure to air pollution can affect the respiratory system, including impeding the lungs' ability to function due to inflammation and destruction of lung tissue. Air pollution also damages the cilia in the nose, leading to sinusitis. Dangerous pollutants to avoid include:

- *Ozone*. The major destructive ingredient in smog. Ozone causes coughing, shortness of breath, and chest pain, and boosts susceptibility to sinus infection.
- *Sulfur dioxide*. Another component of smog, created when sulfur-containing fuel is burned. Sulfur dioxide irritates the airways and constricts the air passages, causing asthma attacks. For those with sinus problems, it can be particularly harmful, as it can suppress mucociliary action.
- *Nitrogen dioxide*. Produced when fuel is burned, especially in motor vehicles and power plants. Nitrogen dioxide contributes to ozone formation and causes bronchitis and an increased chance of sinus infection.
- *Carbon monoxide*. An odorless, colorless gas that comes mainly from automobiles and other combustion exhaust. Carbon monoxide reduces oxygen levels in the blood, starving the body's cells.

To protect yourself from air pollution, be aware of news reports that tell when pollution levels are high, and avoid going outdoors during this time. If you must leave your home or office, avoid strenuous activity and long-term exposure.

- Keep your home well ventilated for at least forty-eight hours after the installation of new carpeting. Potentially harmful volatile organic compounds (VOCs) are released into the air from new carpets.
- Avoid household products (cleaning agents, pesticides, and paints) that are dangerous or that may trigger respiratory problems.
- Avoid aerosol sprays, scented lipsticks, perfumes, talcum powder, room deodorizers, nail polish and remover, and other sources of strong odors.
- Avoid inhaling diesel fumes.
- Test your home for radon—a colorless, odorless gas and powerful carcinogen.
- Avoid all cosmetics and personal-care products that have added perfume or scents.

Strategy 7: Notice Weather Changes

There are many changes in weather that trigger sinus irritation or swelling, including cold air, wind, dry air, humidity, and weather fronts. Exposure to cold air has several effects on the sinuses, such as nasal congestion, secretions, and decreased mucociliary clearance.

If you really want to avoid weather-related sinusitis, then stay out of the cold air, wind, and rain.

THE CRUCIAL ROLE OF AVOIDANCE

Avoidance is the *key* to controlling symptoms triggered by environmental factors. Steps such as staying away from cleaning chemicals or perfumes, avoiding touching the cat or dog, and going into another room if someone is smoking should become natural behavioral responses. If your workplace is full of fumes or chemicals that trigger respiratory distress, ask your employer to move you to another office or consider changing jobs.

Remember, no one can do it for you. Once you understand your disease, as well as the specific allergens and triggers that cause symptoms in your respiratory system, it is vital to use the proactive steps recommended for better breathing.

BEING PROACTIVE FOR CLEARER BREATHING

No matter what the air quality in your home or workplace, it is time to become proactive for cleaner air. It is important to get rid of as many triggers as you can, then try to keep the others under control. For those who need to reduce exposure to dust mites, mold, and mildew, an excellent consumer's site on the Internet is www.allergybuyersclub.com. This site gives timely evaluations of allergy products and rates the best ones.

By learning the exact environmental irritants that trigger your sinus problem, and taking aggressive steps to avoid them, you can reduce your symptoms, and your breathing and quality of life will greatly improve.

Chapter 8

STEP 5:
BOOST HEALING NUTRIENTS

*I can drink one glass of milk, and within a few hours, I
have sinus drainage in the back of my throat. Even when I
was a child, certain foods caused congestion and thick
mucus from my sinuses. Isn't there anything safe to eat for
those with chronic sinusitis?*

—ALAN, *age thirty-six*

Ask any sinus sufferer what triggers the purulent postnasal drip
or headache pain from sinus inflammation, and many will
tell you about an offending food or two, whether milk, meat,
chocolate, cheese, coffee, certain fruits or vegetables, or exotic
spices. Certain foods may make you feel as if the mucus in the
back of your throat is thicker and more difficult to expel. Other
foods can prompt an allergic reaction and subsequent swelling or
even infection.

Still, researchers have tested dietary triggers in various sub-
sets of people with chronic sinus problems without much in the
way of firm conclusions; no doubt this is why many feel science
has largely ignored the food-sinusitis link. There have been

studies that have looked at milk and milk products—eliminating these from patients' diets, then adding the offending food slowly to observe its effect on sinus symptoms. Although researchers doubt that milk makes sinus drainage thicker, most people agree nonetheless that it at least *feels* thicker.

For now there is no good way to predict who should avoid certain foods unless you have a real food allergy. If that is the case, an allergist can guide you in doing the food-elimination diet to find which foods trigger allergic reactions. For sinus sufferers, if you believe a certain food triggers congestion and mucus, leave it out of your diet for two weeks. Then slowly bring it back in—one small bite or sip at a time. Notice any change in sinus symptoms as you do this. By using this elimination method, you may discover your exact offending triggers.

The latest research in the scientific community is focusing not on avoidance but rather on how food can be used to heal your body and promote overall good health, including sinus health. The research emphatically concludes that certain nutrients can boost your body's immune system and lessen, or even ward off, infection.

Nutrients are special compounds found in foods that support your body's repair, growth, and wellness. They include vitamins, minerals, amino acids, essential fatty acids, water, and the calorie sources of carbohydrate, protein, and fat. Some nutrients can be made by the body (nonessential nutrients) and others must come from the diet (essential nutrients). A deficiency of either type of nutrient may lead to illness if left untreated.

In sinusitis, certain nutrients may act as healing mechanisms, even when medications or lifestyle measures have failed. For example, carotenoids found in yellow and orange vegetables, bioflavonoids such as quercetin, and essential fatty acids like flax oil or fish oil block a series of enzymes that are key to mucus production and inflammation. Resveratrol, a natural substance found in peanuts and grapes, may also relieve sinus symptoms by inhibiting certain enzymes called COX (cyclooxygenase) enzymes. COX enzymes make prostaglandins—enzymes of inflammation that produce swelling. Eating these nutrients may help to inhibit these enzymes and improve sinusitis.

FOODS THAT HELP FIGHT SINUS INFECTIONS

For those with sinus problems or respiratory ailments (or any chronic illness, for that matter), healthy nutrition is "fuel" for the body. When you eat a nutritionally well-balanced diet, many other factors fall into place. Good nutrition helps maintain the ventilatory functions of your lungs. Foods that are nutrient dense help fight sinus and respiratory infections and may help to prevent illness. And some foods help you to breathe better, as they heal damaged cilia.

For example, Grandma's steamy chicken soup may be a legitimate medical treatment after all! Chicken soup, also known as Jewish penicillin, is a powerful mucus stimulant. Chicken contains an amino acid called cysteine, which is similar in chemical content to a drug called acetylcysteine. Doctors give acetylcysteine for respiratory infections, such as bronchitis, to help thin mucus, making it easier to expel. Chicken soup helps the cilia of the nose and bronchial passages move quickly so they can defend the respiratory system against contagion.

Drinking hot tea is another natural food treatment that helps to thin mucus and ensure proper hydration of the body.

Super Sinus Food Offenders

While certain foods and nutrients can help to ease sinus inflammation and the resulting mucus buildup, some foods may turn a minor postnasal drip into a major sinus headache. *Cold drinks* are the number-one culprit!

Your *Sinus Cure* rule of thumb: No matter what you drink, do *not* drink it cold. Cold or iced drinks slow the cilia in your sinuses, making it difficult for the mucus to move through. Stagnant mucus and damaged cilia add up to infections, which cause even more damage, as explained on pages 7–9. Avoid all this by refusing *any* iced drinks.

Here are other offending foods you'll want to avoid if you are experiencing sinus problems:

- Alcohol
- Chocolate
- Dairy products
- Food additives
- Sugar
- Yeast

Sipping hot teas made with herbs such as fenugreek, fennel, anise, or sage may help move mucus even more. You don't need medical technology to check whether you are hydrated; just keep drinking until your urine turns light yellow to clear.

Hot, spicy foods also may help you keep mucus thin and flowing. Some of the most potent spicy foods include:

- Cajun spice, made with cayenne peppers, which contain capsaicin, a substance that stimulates nerve fibers and may act as a natural nasal decongestant
- Garlic, an herb that helps to make mucus less sticky
- Horseradish, a root that contains a chemical similar to one found in decongestants

We've found out now iced drinks can paralyze cilia in the sinuses, so what can heal them? *Hot or warm drinks.* Such drinks, *especially hot tea*, heal damaged or slow cilia, helping them to work at clearing mucus out of the sinus cavity. And that can go a long way toward curing sinusitis!

ANTIOXIDANTS GUARD AGAINST INFLAMMATION

Evidence is accumulating that sinusitis and other respiratory diseases may have their origin in deleterious free-radical reactions. Free radicals are the unstable by-products of oxidation, the chemical process that causes iron to rust and a peeled apple or banana to turn brown. In the body, free radicals have one or more unpaired electrons, making them highly reactive, as they tear apart and destroy cell membranes or make cells vulnerable to decay and pathogens. These free radicals damage cells' DNA and mitochondria and leave in their wake inflammation and a depressed immune system.

Over time, there can be an excessive amount of free radicals. This shifts the body's balance in favor of oxidation, termed "oxidative stress," which causes destruction of cellular and tissue function. This oxidation process contributes to a wide variety of

---

Antioxidants and Asthma

A new study from Australia suggests that a diet low in antioxidants may increase asthma symptoms. Researchers put patients with asthma on a diet low in antioxidants for ten days and found that as the levels of antioxidants in the blood dropped, the patients' lung function also decreased and asthma symptoms worsened. Scientists are now testing to see whether increasing antioxidants in the diet can reduce asthma symptoms. Eating a diet filled with fresh fruits, vegetables, and whole grains—all high in antioxidants—is beneficial to your overall health as well as to the health of your respiratory system.

---

disease states, including chronic respiratory problems, infection, and even cancer.

Luckily, certain foods may stop the damage from free radicals. Specifically, some researchers believe that foods rich in antioxidants might help prevent damage in some types of respiratory diseases and boost immune function when a system is under stress—both important benefits for those with chronic sinusitis. *Antioxidants*—beta-carotene and vitamins C and E—are essential nutrients that play a role in the body's cell-protection system and interfere with the disease process by neutralizing free radicals. Antioxidants tie up free radicals and take away their destructive power, perhaps reducing the risk of a number of chronic diseases and even slowing the aging process.

Let's look at some of the most important antioxidants.

Beta-carotene, for Healthy Mucous Membranes

Beta-carotene—found in apricots, carrots, cantaloupe, pumpkin, and spinach—is converted to vitamin A in the body. Vitamin A is crucial for maintaining healthy mucous membranes in your nose, mouth, and lungs. It does this by creating a protective barricade against any invaders, such as viruses or bacteria. Research shows that vitamin A boosts the immune system to help fight off illness and infection, especially viral illness.

The current recommended dietary allowance (RDA) for vitamin A is 5,000 international units (IU) for adults. Vitamin A is found only in foods from animal sources, especially beef, calf, and chicken liver. Dairy products such as milk, butter, cheese, and ice cream are also good sources. Beta-carotene, which is converted to vitamin A, is found in fruits and vegetables. *Caution:* If you take vitamin A supplements, check with your doctor. Too much vitamin A can be toxic. For example, consuming more than 25,000 IU per day in food and supplements increases the risk of toxicity in the body.

Other carotenoid compounds that have antioxidant properties include:

- Alpha-carotene (carrots, cantaloupe, pumpkin)
- Beta-cryptoxanthin (mangoes, nectarines, peaches, tangerines)
- Gamma-carotene (apricots, tomatoes)
- Lycopene (guava, pink grapefruit, tomatoes, watermelon)
- Lutein and zeaxanthin (beets, corn, collard and mustard greens)

Vitamin C, for Its Antihistamine Effect

Vitamin C, also known as ascorbic acid, is a natural sinus booster because of its antihistamine effect. Some people find that taking 1 gram of vitamin C daily helps to lessen inflammation and the subsequent sinus drip. Taking 500 milligrams four times a day may benefit a cold or an allergy. (However, this much vitamin C can also cause stomach upset and diarrhea, so be careful.)

Vitamin C also gives protection against infection and aids in wound healing. Large amounts of vitamin C are used by your body during any kind of healing process, whether it's from a cold, sinus infection, or sinus surgery. When the body is under great stress, the blood levels of ascorbic acid have been found to decline. This decline also occurs with age in both men and women.

Vitamin C plays a vital role in boosting levels of the energizing brain chemical norepinephrine as well. Norepinephrine produces a feeling of alertness and increases concentration, a much-needed boost when sinusitis makes you feel sluggish and fatigued. A deficiency of vitamin C can therefore influence your mood, too, leaving you less attentive.

The current RDA of vitamin C is 90 milligrams for men and 75 milligrams for women, an amount that may be too low to have healing or preventive effect. Talk to your doctor or a certified dietitian to see how much vitamin C may help your situation.

Vitamin E, for Its Ability to Boost Immunity

Vitamin E is important to the body for the maintenance of cell membranes, and this vitamin's antioxidant effect may slow age-related changes of the body. Some studies indicate that vitamin E may help to alleviate respiratory problems while boosting your body's immune function to fight off illness. Vitamin E appears to stimulate the functioning of T cells, which are important powerhouses for fighting disease.

While the RDA for vitamin E is 15 IU for adults, many researchers believe that this amount is too low to prevent disease or have a healing benefit for the body. Because vitamin E is taken in through vegetables and seed oils, it is difficult to ingest larger amounts, especially if you are following a low-fat diet. In fact, to get the 400 IU of vitamin E suggested for prevention of disease, you'd have to eat more than 20,000 calories a day—mostly fat! Not a wise idea.

The Best Sources for Super Sinus Antioxidants

As we now know, much research shows that eating healthful foods, specifically those high in antioxidants (beta-carotene and vitamins C and E) may help. The following is a list of those sources rich in antioxidants. *Note:* When you prepare these foods, *use as little liquid as possible to prevent nutrient loss.* In fact, simply including more raw fruits and vegetables in your diet is the best way to ensure a high intake of healing antioxidants.

Beta-carotene	Vitamin C	Vitamin E
Apricots	Broccoli	Almonds
Asparagus	Cantaloupe	Cod-liver oil
Beef liver	Cauliflower	Corn oil
Broccoli	Kale	Corn oil margarine
Cantaloupe	Kiwi	Hazelnuts
Carrots	Orange juice	Lobster

Beta-carotene	Vitamin C	Vitamin E
Kale	Papaya	Peanut butter
Spinach	Red, green, or yellow peppers	Safflower oil
Sweet potato	Strawberries	Salmon
Watermelon	Sweet potato	Sunflower seeds
Yellow corn	Tomato juice	Walnuts

Healing Foods to Add to Your Diet Each Day

Berries. It is now thought that fruits such as blackberries, blueberries, cranberries, cherries, and raspberries are powerful free radical fighters and healers of the immune system—and the secret is in the color. Anthocyanins (from two Greek words meaning "plant" and "blue") are the universal, water-soluble colorants responsible for the red, purple, and blue hues in many fruits, vegetables, and flowers. More than six hundred anthocyanins have been identified so far, and each fruit and vegetable has a distinct anthocyanin profile. Fruits that are richest in anthocyanins are very strongly colored berries such as the blackberry, blueberry, and bilberry.[1]

Studies show that anthocyanins play an important disease-preventive role in the body by fortifying blood vessel walls. This helps improve blood flow to the tiny blood vessels that keep eyes healthy, as well as to larger blood vessels that help maintain good circulation throughout the body. And these phenolics strengthen collagen, the main part of connective tissue, which is the basis for the structure of skin and all other connective tissue.[2]

In a study published in the journal *Free Radical Research*, scientists compared six berry extracts (wild blueberry, bilberry, cranberry, elderberry, raspberry seed, and strawberry) and a grape seed extract (containing proanthocyanidins) and concluded that edible berries have potent chemopreventive properties. Of the fruits studied, wild bilberry and blueberry extracts possessed the strogest ability to neutralize free radicals, and all fruits were said to impair angiogenesis.[3]

Broccoli. This green, treelike vegetable is full of indoles, isothiocyanates, and sulforaphane—phytochemicals that pack a power punch of healing nutrition! But if you *really* want the highest concentration of these cancer-fighting compounds, get broccoli sprouts at your supermarket in the produce section. The sprouts have ten to one hundred times more sulforaphane than mature broccoli.

Cherries. Cherries contain the compound cyanidin, which is thought to block inflammation enzymes.

Garlic and onions. Garlic and onions increase the sulfur content in the body, which helps in reducing inflammation.

Green and black tea. Tea (green and black) contains a nontoxic chemical, epigallocatechin-3 gallate, that blocks the receptor involved in allergic response. The compounds found in tea help block allergy to pollen, dust, and pets by blocking the production of histamine and IgE. In addition to other benefits, it is reported that drinking five cups of tea a day increases the body's defenses against disease because of a specific chemical called L-theanine. In the liver, L-theanine becomes ethylamine, a molecule that primes the response of an immune blood cell (one of the T cells). These T cells (called gamma delta T cells) prompt the secretion of interferon, a key defense against infection. Also, both green and black teas are naturally rich sources of flavonoids.

Grapes. Trans-resveratrol is a substance produced in the skin of grapes to protect against oxidation and fungal infection caused by external stresses, such as temperature extremes and ultraviolet light. In red wine, trans-resveratrol is found in high concentrations, though its levels vary depending on the particular wine. Studies have identified trans-resveratrol as a powerful antioxidant, more potent than vitamin E and possibly offering disease-preventing protection.

Oranges. Oranges have the flavonoid nobiletin, which may have an anti-inflammatory action. Hesperidin, another flavonoid, is found in the thin orange portion of the citrus peel. Hesperidin may also reduce inflammation.

THE IMPORTANCE OF PROTEIN

Protein is important to build and repair body tissue and fight infection. Immune system powerhouses, like antibodies and T cells, are made up of protein. The only way they "rev up" to protect you from sinus infections is if you replenish their supply. Conversely, too little protein in the diet may lead to symptoms of fatigue, weakness, apathy, and poor immunity.

The average-sized adult needs 45 to 55 grams of protein a day. More protein is needed if there is fever or infection. One ounce of meat, chicken, cheese, or fish provides 7 grams of protein; 1 cup of milk provides 8 grams. Therefore, *5 to 6 ounces of meat per day and 2 cups of milk provide adequate protein for most adults*. For vegetarians, vegetable proteins can make a good substitute for animal protein. An example of this would be to substitute 1½ cups of black beans and rice for a 2-ounce portion of meat. Soy protein and low-fat cottage cheese also are excellent alternative sources.

MINERALS—YOUR SUPER SINUS SAVERS

Not only are vitamins and protein important for healthy sinuses, but there are also some key minerals necessary to boost immune function and fight infection. The best way to ensure the correct balance of these minerals in the body is to obtain them from a variety of food sources, as they can be toxic if taken in larger amounts. Let's take a specific look at the minerals that are important.

Magnesium, for Helping Respiratory Tract Function

Magnesium appears to play a key role in a number of biochemical reactions that are important to respiratory tract function. Recent studies have found that a low intake of magnesium in the diet actually increases bronchial reactivity, resulting in asthma and chronic obstructive airway disease, while magnesium supplementation *reduces* bronchial constriction and may increase the force of the respiratory muscles. As such, magnesium may have a powerful influence by relaxing the airways' smooth muscle and also reducing airway inflammation. Magnesium has been used in the past to treat acute asthma, and there is a belief that in the future magnesium could help to prevent this disease as well. For those with sinusitis, allergies, and asthma, knowing there is hope for this inflammatory condition is exciting news indeed.

The RDA of magnesium is 280 milligrams for women and 350 milligrams for men. Food sources of magnesium include cereals, nuts, tofu, dairy products, bananas, pineapples, plantains, raisins, artichokes, avocados, lima beans, and spinach.

Selenium, for Its Actions as an Antioxidant

The mineral selenium also operates as an antioxidant and protects red blood cells from accumulating hydrogen peroxide, a type of free radical produced by leukocytes, certain white blood cells that may destroy other cells in your body. Vitamin E (see pages 197–198) appears to work positively with selenium in this capacity.

The RDA is 55 micrograms for women and 70 micrograms for men. Foods high in selenium include seafood, liver, and grains from selenium-rich soil.

Zinc, to Help You Resist Infection

Zinc also has antioxidant effects and is vital to the body's resistance to infection and for tissue repair. In fact, long-term infection in the body is associated with zinc deficiency. Some studies suggest that sucking on zinc gluconate lozenges at the start of a cold may lessen its severity. In fact, one study at Dartmouth College reported that students who took zinc lozenges at the onset of a cold had only five days of symptoms, compared with nine days for students who received placebos. This may be because zinc has an antiviral effect in the mouth and nose. Researchers from Wayne State University School of Medicine have suggested that zinc fosters immunity; the body may be unable to fight infection without sufficient supplies of the nutrient.

The RDA for zinc is 12 milligrams for women and 15 milligrams for men. Foods high in zinc include oysters (the richest source), red meats, shrimp, crab, legumes (especially lima beans, black-eyed peas, pinto beans, soybeans, and peanuts), whole grains, miso, tofu, brewer's yeast, cooked greens, mushrooms, green beans, and pumpkin seeds. High doses of zinc are toxic and may, in fact, suppress the immune function, so check with your physician or a certified dietitian for what is safe in your situation.

OTHER KEY HEALING NUTRIENTS

Many health researchers lean toward the premise that specific foods act like medicine—managing, treating, or even preventing chronic conditions. In this regard what you eat may boost good health—or take away from your healthy state. Let's look at even more healing nutrients that will help keep your sinuses in top condition.

Flavonoids, for a Powerful Immune Boost

Flavonoids (or bioflavonoids) include about four thousand compounds that are responsible for the colors of fruits and flowers. Hosts of experiments on bioflavonoids found in the soft white skin of citrus fruits have suggested that these key nutrients increase immune system activation. These biochemically active substances accompany vitamin C in plants and act as antioxidants. You can find bioflavonoids in citrus fruits, green peppers, carrots, berries, squash, apples, grapes, cherries, eggplant, and tomatoes. Tea, red wine, and parsley are also good sources.

QUERCETIN, TO REDUCE INFLAMMATION

Quercetin is a member of a class of nutrients known as bioflavonoids. This powerful anti-inflammatory compound reduces inflammation associated with allergies by stabilizing cell membranes, preventing them from releasing histamine (see page 29). Quercetin also helps prevent the lungs, nasal passages, and eyes from swelling after allergen exposure. This highly concentrated form of bioflavonoid is found in citrus fruits, apples, tomatoes, red and yellow onions, scallions, and broccoli.

SUPPLEMENTING YOUR DIET TO EASE SINUS MISERY

"Wait a minute! I don't think I eat enough nutrients to make a difference in my sinus condition. What do I do now?" If your diet is lacking in nutritional foods, you may want to consider supplementation.

Vitamin Supplements

If you want to take a vitamin to get the nutrients that are missing from your diet, it's smart to start with a multiple vitamin that has the recommended dietary allowances, as suggested by the American Dietetics Association. Then talk with a registered/licensed nutritionist about your specific needs for further vitamins and minerals. If you have chronic sinus infections, you may need to make some dietary changes, but seek advice from professionals first. Also, ask your doctor if the following safe dose ranges recommended by the American Medical Association's

Council on Scientific Affairs would be appropriate for your situation. These recommendations are higher than the ROA, but appear to be safe.

Vitamin A	250 IU to 2,500 IU
Vitamin D	Up to 400 IU (up to age eighteen)
	Up to 200 IU (adults)
Vitamin E	6 IU to 30 IU
Thiamine	1 mg to 2 mg
Riboflavin	1 mg to 2 mg
Vitamin B_6	1.5 mg to 2.5 mg
Folic acid	100 mcg to 250 mcg
Vitamin B_{12}	3 mg to 10 mg
Vitamin C	50 mg to 100 mg

Nutritional Supplements

Dietary supplements include a host of natural products that contain vitamins, minerals, herbs, and amino acids, as well as natural enzymes, organ tissues, metabolites, extracts, or concentrates. For example, *papaya enzymes* are considered a natural supplement. Many doctors recommend papaya enzymes as a natural remedy for reducing the inflammation associated with sinusitis. In fact, chewable papaya enzyme tablets, available without a prescription at your pharmacy or health food store, may help to ease your stuffy sinuses or even ear or throat problems. While these tablets are usually sold for digestion problems, they have been found to be helpful for Eustachian tube blockage (blocked ears), swollen throat, and even hoarseness.

Papaya is also very high in vitamin C, a powerful antioxidant. It has a high carotenoid content and is a good source of dietary fiber and folate.

When using this alternative treatment, take one tablet four times a day and melt it in the mouth between the cheek and the gums. Once dissolved in the mouth, the papaya tablets are absorbed into the circulation and help to reduce swelling and speed healing. If you have an infected, swollen tonsil that is not clearing despite taking an antibiotic, adding the papaya tablet can shrink the tonsil so that the concentration of antibiotic and good white cells is greater. It opens up the area between the cells, decreasing swelling and allowing the antibiotic to enter.

If your Eustachian tube (between the nose and the ear) is blocked, papaya tablets not only reduce swelling of the tube but also liquefy the mucus in the tube. This allows tiny hairs (cilia) to beat and clear the ear. In many bronchial conditions, swelling of membranes is reduced, and the cilia can beat better and clear the bacteria and phlegm.

Because pain in the sinus cavity is always related to swollen membranes, taking papaya enzyme tablets, dissolved buccally, is extremely effective in reducing the swelling and thereby the pain.

Bromelain, a natural protein-digesting enzyme that helps to reduce inflammation, is available as a supplement and is a key factor in sinusitis and allergic diseases. Bromelain inhibits the release of certain inflammation-causing chemicals and also activates a chemical in the blood and tissues that breaks down fibrin, a protein-sugar complex that is partly responsible for blood clotting. By breaking down fibrin, bromelain reduces swelling. That's because fibrin prevents injured tissues from draining, and when they can't drain, they swell. Bromelain is available in tablet or capsule form for supplementation use. It is also found in pineapple.

Clear•Ease is a tablet containing 1 million enzyme units of bromelain and 500,000 enzyme units of papain (papaya), buccal (melt in the mouth) administration. Take three times daily.

Essential Fatty Acids, to Decrease Inflammation

Anyone with sinus disease knows that inflammation is something you do *not* want! Essential fatty acids (EFAs) are not manufactured by the body, but they *are* essential to sinus health because they reduce the swelling (and pain) associated with allergic response. They work by aiding in the production of prostaglandins that counter inflammation.

EFAs are available in oils containing omega-3 (fish oils), as well as in oils containing omega-6 (linolenic acid and gamma-linolenic acid [GLA]), which are found in plant oils such as evening primrose, black currant, and borage.

You find omega-3 in oily kinds of fish, such as anchovy, bluefish, capelin, dogfish, herring, mackerel, salmon, sardines, shad, sturgeon, tuna, and whitefish. Or take fish oil capsules, which may reduce inflammation that stems from arthritis. These fatty acids enable the body to make more products that tend to decrease the inflammation. The fish oil eicosapentaenoic acid (EPA) is available in capsules without a prescription at your drugstore or health food store. (It is also possible to get this amount simply by making fish an important part of your diet.) It takes twelve to sixteen weeks of omega-3 therapy before benefits begin.

Some patients with sinusitis, allergy, and asthma have found improvement in symptoms when they take fish oil capsules for a few months. But it is important to use fish oil as a supplement to your doctor's prescribed regimen, not instead of it. When used in the doses suggested on the label, no serious side effects are known.

Breakfast in Bed?

If you suffer from early morning sneezing and choking on thick postnasal drip, try having breakfast in bed. In sleep the body temperature is lowered, and the cilia that defend the body do less work, so dust accumulates in your nasal passages. On awakening, the body wants to get rid of that dust and at the same time warm itself. So, especially if you are allergic, you sneeze and cough. This certainly warms the body, but then a "cascade" starts that is hard to stop. To avoid the initial morning sneezing, have hot tea before you get out of bed. You can keep it warm overnight in a thermos or on a hot plate—or it can be offered to you in the morning by a loving mate. It will reduce the morning symptoms.

Note: Vegetarians who want to gain the anti-inflammatory benefit associated with essential fatty acids can take borage seed oil, flaxseeds, flaxseed oil, or evening primrose oil. All of these are known to be helpful in offsetting inflammation.

WHAT TO WATCH OUT FOR IN YOUR FOODS

Sulfites, which are used in foods and drugs as preservatives, can cause fatal allergic reactions in some people, many of whom also suffer from sinusitis. Such sulfites as bisulfite, potassium metabisul-

---

Foods That often Contain Tartrazine
(FD&C Yellow No. 5)

- Certain breakfast cereals
- Cake mixes
- Commercial pies
- Commercial gingerbread
- Chocolate chips
- Butterscotch chips
- Commercial frostings
- Ready-to-eat canned puddings
- Certain instant and regular puddings
- Certain ice creams and sherbets
- Certain candy coatings
- Candy drops and hard candies
- Colored marshmallows
- Flavored carbonated beverages
- Flavored drink mixes

---

fite, sodium bisulfite, and sodium sulfite are frequently contained in bakery products, dehydrated potatoes, corn syrup, shellfish, salad dressings, pickles, wine and beer, and dried fruits. Surprisingly, sulfites are also found in some prescription and nonprescription drugs used by those with breathing problems, including epinephrine and some nebulizers.

Some artificial colors, particularly tartrazine or yellow food dye number 5, can be dangerous for those with allergies or asthma. Yellow food dye number 5 might create breathing prob-

Common Foods That May Contain Sulfiting Agents

- Restaurant salads (lettuce, tomatoes, carrots, peppers, and dressings)
- Fresh fruit
- Dried fruits (such as apricots)
- Wine, beer, and cordials
- Alcohol as well as all sparkling grape juices (including those that are nonalcoholic)
- Potatoes (such as french fries and chips)
- Sausage meats (especially those made outside of the United States)
- Cider and vinegar
- Pickles
- Dehydrated vegetables
- Cheese and cheese mixtures

lems for those who have asthma and those who are allergic to aspirin. Products containing *iodine*, such as table salt, can also wreak havoc with your sinuses or respiratory system if you are allergic to it.

If you are allergic to *molds*, certain foods may exacerbate your problem. Watch out for fermented foods (such as beer, cider, sauerkraut, vinegar, and wine) as well as foods made with yeast (such as breads, rolls, and many bakery products). Cheese, sour cream, buttermilk, and mushrooms can also aggravate a mold allergy.

Common Food Allergens

- Alcohol (such as wine containing sulfites or other allergens)
- Berries (usually blueberries, raspberries, and strawberries)
- Eggs
- Fish (usually shellfish and whitefish)
- Grains (commonly wheat, gluten, corn, and rye)
- Milk proteins (can also cause lactose intolerance)
- Peanuts
- Peppers
- Soy
- Yeast

BOOSTING IMMUNE POWER THROUGH HEALING FOODS!

Eating healing foods filled with special nutrients is important to halt and reverse sinus symptoms. There are no absolute guarantees that the nutrients you eat will "cure" your sinusitis. However, the latest research points toward good nutrition as a vital part of coping with the symptoms and boosting your immune system so you can fight infection and disease.

Chapter 9

STEP 6: DE-STRESS TO STAY WELL

It never fails. As soon as tax season starts, I face an on-slaught of sinus infections. I stay up too late, wake up before dawn, miss meals, and have horrible anxiety that I won't meet the IRS deadline for my clients. Then the sinus problems begin. Every time I get overextended and run-down, I become a prime candidate for sinus infection!

—ANNE, CPA, age forty-seven

Stress, and the resulting negative emotional and physical consequences, may be contributing factors to acute sinus infections or even chronic sinusitis. Keeping infections at bay is directly related to the functioning of a *strong* immune system. With a depleted immune system, the body is at risk of being overwhelmed by invading bacteria and viruses, resulting in weeks of suffering.

When you are living with sinusitis, your stress level is already high. Not only do you face everyday stress from family or work, but you also face the stress of not breathing through your nose, constant sinus headaches, and infections that cause fever and body aches.

But what *is* stress? In simplest terms stress is a response of the body to any demand. It is a biological phenomenon that affects both the central and autonomic nervous systems, as well as the endocrine and immune systems. And it is a key contributing factor to illness, including heart disease, depression, anxiety disorders, asthma and allergy, and even sinus infections.

STRESS AND YOUR IMMUNE SYSTEM

As you probably realize, there is an extremely close relationship between your inner attitude and daily thoughts and the effect these have on your body and mind. This mind-body interaction is called psychoneuroimmunology, or PNI, and a tremendous amount of research is being conducted in this field to determine the connection between stress, emotions, and disease.

How Your Mind Influences Your Body

Psychoneuroimmunology means mind-body interplay. *Psycho* stands for mind, *neuro* for the neuroendocrine system (the nervous and hormonal systems), and *immunology* for the immune system. Those on the cutting edge of psychoneuroimmunology contend that many influences are at work in each of us to either keep us well or allow us to get sick. Scientific evidence suggests that factors such as stress, negative feelings, and lack of social support can influence both immune status and function as well as lead to the onset and progression of disease. Although research is still in the early stages, findings to date also suggest that psychological factors play a role in autoimmune diseases such as allergies, arthritis, and multiple sclerosis.

The Damaging Factor of Daily Hassles

While there is still some controversy regarding the connection between stress and sinus problems, there are theories that suggest it is the annoying *daily* hassles—chronic stress—that greatly affect you and your symptoms. Especially when coupled with chronic sinus symptoms and disturbed sleep, this psychological stress may heighten your reaction to your sinus problem and increase the chances that your mind will dwell on its symptoms.

Chronic stress persists for weeks or even months, and produces cortisol, the body's main stress-induced hormone. When cortisol becomes elevated and remains that way for an extended period of time, it damages the cells that comprise your immune system. As a result of being bathed in the stress-related chemicals, the immune system is no longer capable of keeping infections or diseases at bay. So the invading virus or bacterium proliferates to the point where it infects many cells, eventually leading to symptoms and increased chance of illness.

Exposure to the invaders normally would have resulted in no problems, provided your immune system was strong. It is as a result of the chronic stress you were under that your immune system did not work at full capacity to overwhelm the invaders.

The effect of stress on immune function has been studied worldwide. For instance, researchers at Ohio State University studied the immune systems of people who cared for loved ones with Alzheimer's disease to see the effects of chronic stress. These scientists found that the ongoing stress of caring for someone with Alzheimer's depressed the caregiver's immune system even *two years* after the patient had died! Another revealing study was done on forty-five male medical students who were taking final exams to see if stress negatively affected their resistance to disease. Specifically these students were studied three to four weeks prior to exams, then again during exams, to see how they responded to a hepatitis vaccine. Compared to students who received the vaccine under unstressed conditions, the stressed students showed much weaker immune responses (as measured by the levels of natural killer cells).

It is interesting that an increase in respiratory problems in young children has been strongly associated with starting primary school. This is undoubtedly related to the many infectious agents to which the children are exposed upon entering school. Yet researchers have also found that salivary cortisol—as you recall, cortisol increases in response to stress—is significantly increased during the week before children begin kindergarten and for the first week of school.

When cortisol becomes extremely elevated, as with chronic stress, and remains so for an extended period of time, it can actually inhibit the lymphocytes, or white blood cells. Other chemicals produced by the brain's autopilot—known as the autonomic nervous system—can similarly damage the cells that comprise the immune system.

TAKING CONTROL OF THE STRESS YOU FEEL

With the breakthrough research currently being done in the field of psychoneuroimmunology (mind-body interplay), no one can deny that stress negatively affects immune function and your symptoms. Yet you *do* have control. Starting today, you can begin to control unhealthy reactions due to stress, if you follow the suggestions presented in this section.

Step 1: Evaluating Your Stress Level

The problem with stress is not the stressor itself. Rather, it is *our personal reaction* to the stress. Experts claim that the stressor represents 10 percent of the problem as we see it; the other 90 percent is our *reaction* to this. When we are exposed to a stressful situation perceived as threatening, our bodies prepare for confrontation. This physical response, known as the "fight or flight" response, is controlled by our hormones and nervous system and dates back to prehistoric times, as early humans prepared to fight or flee their attackers. Although we do not live in the age of fighting wild animals anymore, those "wild animals" are constantly there in such forms as disputes with our boss, a phone that won't quit ringing, and a whining, persistent child.

For those with chronic sinus problems, sometimes the "wild animal," or stressor, is the unending congestion, headache pain, or sleepless nights. For example, when you begin to get a pounding sinus headache right before an important meeting at work, your body produces adrenaline. This release of adrenaline is like sending a thousand messages to various key parts of the body at once, resulting in a racing heart, increased blood pressure, and a system on red alert. These messages prepare your body to deal with the stress or pain.

Because stress can show itself through a wide variety of physical changes and emotional responses, it is important to identify these feelings. Stress symptoms vary greatly from one person to the next, and learning to identify the ways in which

Some Early Warning Signs of Stress

- Anger
- Anxiety
- Back pain
- Body aches and pains
- Boredom
- Bossiness
- Change in bowel or bladder habits
- Compulsive eating or gum chewing
- Constant worrying
- Crying
- Dizziness
- Dry mouth
- Excessive smoking
- Feeling of doom
- Forgetfulness
- Headaches and other aches
- Inability to make decisions
- Increased use of drugs, alcohol, or cigarettes
- Indigestion
- Lack of creativity
- Light-headedness
- Loneliness
- Loss of sense of humor
- Memory loss
- Palpitations
- Racing heart
- Restlessness

- Ringing in the ears
- Sleep problems
- Sweaty palms
- Teeth grinding
- Unhappiness

your body and mind show stress is an important step in treating and managing this disease. Check the accompanying box for early warning signs and symptoms of stress, and see which ones you may have experienced.

Whatever your problems with sinus disease, too much stress does *not* have to be a contributing factor. You can learn to manage your stress just as you manage other areas of your life, and in doing so, you will reduce the symptoms of this common malady.

Step 2: Identifying and Removing the Source of Stress in Your Life

The main strategy in dealing with stress is to identify and remove or reduce the source. If your stress is from overwork, learn to delegate at your office or at home. If your stress is from overextending yourself with outside commitments, rethink how to modify your priorities and put this plan into action.

As you seek to minimize stress, ask yourself the following:

- What stressors can I eliminate in my life?
- What stressors can I avoid?

■ Of the stressors that remain, how can I reduce their
  intensity or manage them?

■ What strategies do I need to use to make these changes?

*Setting priorities and budgeting your time each day is the first step
in gaining balance in your life.* And having a balanced life can
help you deal with life's stressors more effectively.

But before you start reorganizing your life, let's do a reality
check. The reality is that there are only twenty-four hours in
each day—no more, no less. Of those twenty-four hours, depending on how much you sleep, you have available to you
about sixteen hours of actual awake time. So here's how to effectively balance and de-stress your days:

List all commitments. Make a list of all the commitments you
have each week. Then check off those that are most essential.
Include your current obligations, such as work, family commitments, and community involvement. Also include time for personal needs, such as exercise, rest, and relaxation. When you
start adding to your list a host of volunteer commitments, evening meetings, career obligations, or other activities, you could
face an overload, resulting in additional stress. To de-stress, you
need to pick and choose where to draw the line—and no one
can draw this line but *you*.

Make a weekly schedule. Schedule your week for peak ef-
ficiency. Staying employed is a major commitment for most
people. However, is it necessary to bring work home each
night, work late at night, or go into the office on the week-
end? On your schedule jot down time for meditation, exercise, and enjoyable activities such as being with friends and
family.

Make vital choices. Be selective about your commitments. Keep the ones that are most important to your health and your family's well-being. If you can't keep them, what changes do you need to make in your list of priorities? Work on what you can change, and accept what you can't—just be sure to stay on top of the time spent on *all* commitments so that your main priorities get done each day.

Stay focused. Number the items in order of their priority to you. This will help you to stay focused on what you need to do each day and work on the items that must receive your attention first. Some people find that crossing off each item as they complete it gives them a sense of accomplishment. Divide large tasks that seem overwhelming into several days. Again, write down time *for yourself.* Without this downtime, it is virtually impossible to recharge.

Be realistic. A constant push for perfection can cause undue stress, which results in burnout. Make sure your to-do list each week is balanced and reasonable, and does *not* put you into overload.

Step 3: Using Stress Reduction Tools Each Day

Once you have identified the sources of stress in your life, it's time to take charge and eliminate the dangerous symptoms through stress reduction tools. In order for the following methods to work, you must make time daily to relax, unwind, exercise, and replace your high anxiety with a soothing sense of calm.

EXERCISE FOR THIRTY MINUTES A DAY

You've probably given every reason in the book for *not* exercising, including:

■ How can I exercise when I get a splitting sinus headache every time my foot pounds the pavement?

■ Sure, I'd exercise if I had some energy. The medication the doctor gave me makes me so tired, it's all I can do to function at work!

■ Exercise? I can't even breathe through my nose. Why would I think of exerting more pressure on my body?

■ Sorry, just thinking about exercising makes me depressed. . . .

■ If you would eliminate my sinus congestion and head pain, then maybe I'd feel like exercising.

No matter what your excuse or how out of shape you may be, exercise *is* considered to be the best way to reduce the deleterious effects of stress. Exercise has been proved to have many benefits, including:

■ Boosting energy
■ Combating weight gain
■ Improving physical status and disease symptoms
■ Enhancing psychological contentment
■ Decreasing anxiety and depression

"Why does walking for thirty minutes or riding the exercise bike during the evening news reduce stress symptoms?" you might ask. *Because exercise helps to restore the body's neurochemical balance, which affects our emotional state.* Not only does physical activity increase alpha waves, which are associated with relaxation and meditation, but exercise also acts as a displacement defense mechanism for those who are literally "stressed out."

If you have ever participated in a lengthy period of aerobics or walked for several miles, perhaps you know the benefit of this displacement defense mechanism. Isn't it difficult to worry about daily stressors when you are working so hard physically? Your mind is focused on the activity . . . not on the problems you face each day. It makes sense that if you are more in control of your life after exercise, then out-of-control situations that cause chronic stress are less likely to affect you.

That evening walk may clear your head from sinus congestion and pain. In fact, physical exercise drains sinuses in two ways:

1. As you move around more, the blood supply in your nostrils increases.
2. The added blood supply floods your nose with thin mucus, helping to push out the stagnant, bacteria-laden mucus that's making you feel miserable.

Exercise also acts as "nature's decongestant." Your body produces adrenaline, which shrinks swollen blood vessels all around the body and particularly in your nose.

Some of the best exercises for increasing sinus drainage while also decreasing stress symptoms include:

- Walking
- Bicycling
- Bowling
- Dancing
- Karate
- Aerobics
- Stair climbing

- Strength training
- Tae kwon do

Caution: If you are older than thirty-five, get a medical doctor's consent before engaging in any exercise program. Sometimes medications taken for sinus or respiratory problems can increase heart rate during exercise. Also, swimming may not be the best exercise for those with sinusitis or allergies, especially if the chlorine in the pool irritates your nasal passages.

LEARN TAI CHI FOR MIND-BODY HEALTH

Tai chi (or tai chi chuan, as it is known in China) is an ancient Chinese defensive martial art that is similar to shadowboxing. With tai chi you follow a series of slow, graceful movements that mimic the movements you do in daily life.

The various movements require you to move forward, backward, and from side to side in a carefully coordinated manner—flowing together in harmony, as though your body were doing one continuous movement.

Tai chi is based on the theory that continuous practice will help train the body to respond quickly in a crisis. Since the movements emphasize complete relaxation and passive concentration, they can be compared with "meditation in motion," which is said to be healing to the nervous system. The gentle, graceful movements, along with deep breathing patterns, are said to lower blood pressure and heart rate.

For centuries in China, tai chi was a secret heritage among the people and was taught by one generation to the next. It became increasingly popular in the twentieth century and now is practiced worldwide.

Tai chi speeds healing, improves circulation, boosts immune function, and decreases stress. The exercise emphasizes deep abdominal breathing, which could help in maintaining better lung function. As it's a low-impact exercise, it is perfect for older people or those who have severe breathing difficulties. It increases the heart rate and helps to improve overall cardiovascular function.

According to clinical research, tai chi may provide an added benefit, especially to elderly people, in warding off age-related breathing problems. In a study reported in the *Journal of the American Geriatrics Society*, tai chi was found to help improve lung function in older people.

To learn this discipline, hire a private tai chi instructor or purchase a book or video on tai chi. Or you may enjoy doing this in the company of others at a local health spa or YMCA. Many proponents of tai chi find that doing it once a day is adequate to receive its relaxing and toning benefits.

TRY YOGA TO RELIEVE STRESS

Yoga is a classical Indian practice that is built on the foundation of ethics (*yama*) and personal discipline (*niyama*). It is used to relieve stress, achieve mind-body connectedness, and heal the body.

Because yoga is a type of mind-body therapy, the postures or movements are structured to stretch the mind and body beyond their normal limits, then make them act in unison again. Using deep breathing, concentration techniques, and body poses, you learn to calm your mind and increase flexibility and strength. *Pranayama*, which is the conscious focus on and control of breath to heal disease, is an important part of yoga.

Yoga comes from the Sanskrit word meaning "union" and

goes back as far as five thousand years. The many postures of yoga can relieve mild aches and pains, increase flexibility and co-ordination, reduce stress, and promote deep relaxation. Breathing exercises done with different yoga positions can increase blood circulation. Yoga may also be helpful with some respiratory problems. It not only provides the benefit of relaxing your body, but the various positions can also help to improve your breathing and ease the expectoration of mucus.

Learning yoga can cost as little as $10 through purchasing a "how-to" book or an instructional video, or you can join a yoga class at your local gym or YMCA for a monthly rate. To experience optimum results, practice daily yoga in the form of meditation and postures.

DECREASE YOUR INTAKE OF CAFFEINE

Studies show that 80 percent of Americans regularly consume caffeine. Of this number many people tell of "craving" caffeine and suffer withdrawal symptoms when they give it up. While earlier we discussed caffeine as a natural remedy for breathing problems (see pages 149–150), it is also the *only food ingredient* that can *increase* your stress level. It does that by mimicking the stress response—that is, by increasing blood pressure and heart rate and acting as a stimulant. Most of us get our caffeine from coffee, but it is also found in tea, soda, chocolate, and some over-the-counter pain relievers.

As you work to de-stress, read the labels of food products and medications to spot caffeine and eliminate it from your diet.

BREAK THE CYCLE OF ANXIETY

Irrespective of the sinus symptom—headache, toothache, postnasal drip, earache, or cough—you can suffer from a heightening of symptoms by a process known as *anxiety reinforcement*. For example, the more it hurts, the more you tense up; the more anxious you feel, the more tense you get, and the more it hurts. It is absolutely essential to break the anxiety reinforcement cycle, whatever the illness.

The easiest way to do so is through breathing and biofeedback. Normally you inhale and exhale equally but, when anxious, you take shorter, faster breaths. Inhalation takes longer than exhalation. When you breathe in, the diaphragm and the chest muscles contract; on exhalation the diaphragm and the chest muscles relax.

To relax, try to stay in the exhalation state longer than in the inhalation state. Breathe in to the count of four and out to the count of six. As you exhale, let that be a signal to relax the whole body. Raise your hand or finger as you exhale, count to three, and at the count of three drop the finger and let that be a signal to relax the jaw and body.

Use a mirror as your personal biofeedback machine. Watch your face as it relaxes. The more you see the face and jaw relax, the more correctly you are doing it. Remember, you cannot feel anxiety if your muscles are relaxed. Some people find that wearing a watch helps them remember to practice this form of breathing control each hour.

USE MUSIC THERAPY AFTER A STRESSFUL DAY

Music therapy is an excellent nonpharmacological way to reduce anxiety, stress, or grief. Matching their creative and musical prowess with the latest results from laboratory studies, researchers and composers are turning out compositions from classical music to babbling brooks, specifically designed to relax you, reduce mental fatigue, and lower stress.

Music therapy is used for treating various neurological, mental, or behavioral disorders such as developmental and learning disabilities, Alzheimer's disease and other age-related problems, brain injuries, and acute and chronic pain. Still, you can use music therapy simply to calm down after a stressful day. If you have difficulty maintaining sleep because your active mind is running in high gear, composer and researcher Steven Halpern says that certain musical forms can transport the listener's brain into the alpha wave pattern, a state of relaxation much like meditation. One way to begin is to tune your radio to an easy-listening music station. Or start playing your favorite CD of classical music. Make sure the tempo is slow and rhythmic in order to lull you to relaxation, then sleep.

LET DEEP MUSCLE RELAXATION CALM YOU DOWN

Your body responds to tense thoughts or unpleasant situations with muscle tension, which can cause pain or discomfort. Deep muscle relaxation reduces the muscle tension as well as any anxiety you feel. It involves mindfully concentrating on different muscle groups as you contract, then relax, all the major muscle groups in the body. You begin with the head, neck, and upper arms, then progress down to the chest, back, stomach, pelvis, legs, and feet.

To do this exercise, focus on each set of muscles. For example, focus on your facial muscles and tense these muscles to the count of ten. Then release to the count of ten. Next do your jaw muscles, then your neck and upper arms, and proceed until you reach the tips of your toes.

Use deep abdominal breathing along with progressive muscle relaxation for the ultimate stress reducer—*and* to help the body prepare for sound sleep.

ENGAGE IN THE RELAXATION RESPONSE ANYTIME

The relaxation response offers a real potential to reduce emotional, negative thoughts—and increase your ability to self-manage stress. It is done by developing an inner quiet and peacefulness, calming one's negative thoughts and worries, and finding a mental focus apart from your worries.

Set aside a period of about twenty minutes that you can devote to this practice of relaxation. Remove outside distractions that can disrupt your concentration: turn off the radio, the television, and even the ringer on the telephone if need be. Lie flat on a bed or the floor, or recline comfortably so that your whole body is supported, relieving as much tension or tightness in your muscles as you can. Use a pillow or cushion under your head if this helps.

During the twenty-minute period, remain as still as you can; try to focus your thoughts as much as possible on the immediate moment, and eliminate any outside thoughts that may compete for your attention. As you go through these steps, in your own way try to imagine that every muscle in your body is now becoming loose, relaxed, and free of any excess tension. Picture all of your muscles beginning to unwind; imagine them beginning to go loose and limp. Concentrate on making your breathing even. As you exhale, picture your muscles becoming even more relaxed, as if you were somehow breathing the tension away. At the end of twenty minutes, take a few moments to study and focus on the feelings and sensations you have been able to achieve. Notice whether areas that felt tight and tense at first now feel more loose and relaxed and whether any areas of tension or tightness remain.

Benefits of the Relaxation Response

The relaxation response slows down the sympathetic nervous system, leading to:

- Decreased heart rate
- Decreased blood pressure
- Decreased sweat production
- Decreased oxygen consumption
- Decreased production of catecholamines (brain chemicals associated with the stress response)
- Decreased production of cortisol (stress hormone)

GET A MASSAGE TO REDUCE MUSCLE TENSION

When you are very stressed and your muscles are tense, they build up lactic acid. This makes the muscles even more tense, but massage may help relieve this.

Studies released from the University of Miami School of Medicine's Touch Research Center found that the benefits of massage include heightened alertness, relief from depression and anxiety, an increase in the number of natural "killer cells" in the immune system, lower levels of the stress hormone cortisol, and less difficulty in getting to sleep. Another study reported that patients who received massage for pain-related ailments took fewer narcotics or sedatives for the pain—an important benefit for those with constant sinus pain. The patients also reported a decreased heart rate, a drop in blood pressure, and even a lower skin temperature. Unlike any medications taken for the same problems, massage has no negative side effects.

Massage therapists can be found everywhere from health spas and gyms to physicians' and chiropractors' offices. Neuromuscular and sports/injury massage therapists specialize in relief of muscle pain and may often work in medical settings. Check the credentials of the massage therapist you use to make sure he or she is certified and licensed (L.M.T.).

DAYDREAM YOUR TROUBLES AWAY

Visualization (or guided imagery) is a stress release activity that you can do wherever you are, any time of the day or night. This exercise is very similar to daydreaming. Using visualization or imagery, allow your imagination to take over as you focus on your senses to create a desired state of relaxation in your mind.

Throughout history, there have always been "healing" places—places where people traveled to find health and solace. The Greeks had great temples; the Europeans had the hot water baths; and the Native Americans had the hot springs. The reason these places worked to encourage natural healing is that they allowed the person a time to rest. When someone, say, with asthma arrived exhausted, the person was immediately put to bed, made to rest, and given plain foods that were easy to digest. With the bed rest and relaxation, his or her natural cortisol level had time to recover from the stress of illness and return to normal.

So find a healing place where you can be comfortable, and allow about fifteen minutes for this exercise. Take several deep breaths while sitting or lying down, and close your eyes. Imagine a relaxing place—somewhere you have been before, so it can be clearly visualized in your mind. This might be sitting on the seashore at sunset or sunrise, at a mountain cabin next to a babbling brook, or floating on a raft in the lake on a sunny day. Continue to breathe slowly and keep this image in your mind. As you explore your mental picture of your relaxing spot, imagine all the stress, worries, and tension leaving your body.

After about fifteen minutes, slowly open your eyes and acclimate yourself to the surroundings in the room. Stretch your arms and legs; gently move your head from side to side and feel the tension release. Carry this calm feeling with you as you finish your day, or close your eyes for peaceful slumber.

Step 4: Getting Healing Sleep to Boost Immune Function

Sleep is vital to diminish the signs of stress. During the deepest level of sleep, your body is revitalized and tissue damage is repaired. In fact, deep sleep may be the perfect "cure" for ongoing sinus misery, as it restores the body, repairing skin, building bone and muscle, and strengthening the immune system. Studies show that difficulty in sleeping may accentuate the nonspecific aches and pains you feel.

The problem with poor sleep or reduced sleep is that it could possibly result in additional daytime fatigue, causing reduced levels of activity; declining endurance and fitness; and increased aches, pains, and illnesses, such as sinus infections. This can become a vicious cycle that can make you more vulnerable to colds or infection.

To get sounder sleep, you will need to use a combination of steps, including exercise, the right foods, and relaxation strategies. Check out the following suggestions to get an idea of what to include on your list:

■ *Refrain from stimulants and alcohol for at least six hours before bedtime.*

- *Check your medications.* Ask your doctor or pharmacist about your sinus medications to see if they are making it difficult to get sound sleep. Many medications for sinus problems cause insomnia or nervousness, so work with your doctor to find the one that allows you to breathe—and sleep.
- *Avoid naps.* While an occasional nap may help if you are not feeling well, naps can interfere with a good night's sleep. If you do need to nap, try to do so before 2:00 P.M. and make it a brief "catnap."
- *Don't go to bed until you are tired.* Spending less time in bed will allow you to fall asleep faster and get deeper, more efficient sleep.
- *Have a regular wake-up time.* No matter what day it is, try to wake up at the same time regardless of when you went to bed.
- *Use the de-stressing tips to wind down before bedtime.* Turn on soothing music, then read, talk quietly, take a bath or shower, or practice yoga, meditation, or other relaxation techniques. Rituals are important for the expectation and routine they create.
- *Get regular exercise for deeper sleep.* Be sure to stop exercise at least four hours before bedtime or you will be too keyed up to fall asleep. If possible, try to exercise outside to gain the extra benefit of natural sunlight. This will help set your body's natural circadian rhythm, allowing for regular sleep.
- *Make sure your room is quiet enough for deep sleep.* Wear earplugs if you are bothered by noises while sleeping. Some people find that it helps to have "white noise"—either by using a machine that pro-

duces a humming sound or by tuning the radio to a station that has gone off the air.

■ *Eat foods that have a calming effect.* Dr. Judith Wurtman, a nutrition researcher at the Massachusetts Institute of Technology, has found that foods that are high in carbohydrates—such as breads, cereal, pasta, or sherbet—raise the level of serotonin (a mood-elevating chemical) in the brain. When serotonin levels rise, we feel a calming effect and sleep more soundly.

■ *Take a warm bath well before bedtime.* Sleep usually follows the cooling phase of your body's temperature cycle. After your bath keep the temperature in your bedroom cool to see if you can influence this phase.

Step 5: Changing Your Attitude

Attitude is crucial for wellness. Still, let's face it: It's not easy to be positive when you are exhausted from sinusitis or have a pounding headache three days in a row. Nonetheless, you must be positive to de-stress, and the results of a variety of studies now provide mounting evidence that optimism may be one of the missing links for optimal health, as it speeds the production of new immune cells and reduces the levels of the stress hormone cortisol.

In a recent study, researchers found that the blood chemistry of professional actors actually changes during a performance. In one experiment actors alternated between two plays, one happy and one depressing. This staging was repeated several times over a two-week period, during which time researchers took blood samples from the actors after each performance, with astonishing results. They found that simply by *acting* depressed, the actors had actually depressed their immune systems! But when they returned to acting happy, their blood chemistry returned to healthy levels again.

No, you don't have to be a Marlon Brando or Laurence Olivier to be able to summon positive emotions at will. But you may want to practice smiling and seeing life through "rose-colored glasses" if you want to move beyond sinus despair! Study after study shows that negative emotions such as chronic anger, pessimism, mistrust, cynicism, and depression throw the immune system into a state that makes it difficult to resist disease—yes, even sinusitis. Scientists have also found that negative people have burdened their immune system and are more prone to develop certain diseases, then recover more slowly than their positive counterparts.

Whatever stress reduction techniques you need—regular exercise, the relaxation response, or healing sleep—it's important to continue these each day for maximum benefit. Make downtime a daily ritual so you can focus on your personal needs, including sinus health. You will find that your productivity will soar as you feel more rested and relaxed, and the chances are great that your bouts of sinus problems will diminish.

Chapter 10

STEP 7: USE EFFECTIVE MEDICAL THERAPIES

I use an inhaler when my bronchial tubes get inflamed from constant postnasal drip and I become short of breath. When the sinus decongestant keeps me wide awake at night, I have to take a small gray pill to fall asleep.

Ever since childhood I've been plagued with some type of sinus problem, whether it's postnasal drip, thick phlegm in my throat, nasal congestion, or headache. I remember not making the junior high chorus because my voice was so nasal from my swollen sinuses. Then I missed my senior prom because I had a sinus and ear infection with a high fever. My medicines (all eleven of them) are the only thing I have to stay halfway normal.

— JIM, *age thirty-five*

Even though you've learned about the various ways to end or manage sinusitis—including pulsatile nasal irrigation, herbal therapy, changes in diet, improved sleep, and regular exercise—effective medications can be necessary to stay "halfway normal," as Jim, above, says. Medications can give much-needed relief of the various sinus symptoms without causing harmful side effects. These treatment measures often can halt the disease, preventing further damage and deterioration.

A host of specific medications—including expectorants, inhaled and oral decongestants, antihistamines, and inhaled and oral steroids—work separately or in combination to treat or prevent infection, pain, swelling, and other symptoms. Sometimes powerful antibiotics are necessary to stop sinus infections and the subsequent thick, discolored mucus and pain from inflammation. If your sinus disease is persistent and stubborn, cortisone shots or oral steroids may be required to shrink mucous membranes or nasal polyps.

In the past, oral medications used to be the treatment of choice for sinusitis as well as other respiratory diseases. Today inhaled medications that work directly on the airways are frequently prescribed. These medications are convenient and easy to use, and have fewer side effects than oral medications, as most do not enter your system. Yet they do help to reduce swelling and open up the sinus passages. Inhaled steroids are used to keep inflammation down. Newer medication, such as inhaled cromolyn sodium, also plays a role in preventing sinusitis if you have allergies.

The chances are great that by using some of the following medications, along with the other easy recommendations in this book, you can regain control of your sinus problem and enjoy a higher quality of life. After you read the rest of this chapter, talk with your doctor about what might best meet your particular needs.

Medicines Helpful for Sinusitis

Type of Medication	Common Uses
Decongestants	Control nasal stuffiness or congestion
Antihistamines	Control sneezing and drippiness; may relieve congestion from allergy
Anticholinergics	Control running, drippy nose
Steroids	Control all allergy and asthma symptoms
Mast cell stabilizers (cromolyn sodium)	Prevent nasal congestion before exposure to allergens

CURRENT STRATEGIES IN DRUG TREATMENT

What is the most widely used form of medication for sinusitis, along with allergic rhinitis, colds, and a host of other respiratory problems? Decongestants, both oral and inhaled, either over-the-counter or prescription. If your doctor determines that you have an infection, then antibiotics are still the standard mode of treatment, and these differ greatly, from generic brands to name brands—some of which are equally effective and some of which are not.

Decongestants

Decongestants can provide much relief, especially if your sinus passages are swollen and congested. They are used to shrink blood vessels, reduce swelling in the nasal passage, and open the mucous membranes in the nose. The result? You have improved airflow, decreased pressure in the sinuses and head, and subsequently less discomfort. You breathe more clearly—but not without side effects.

Commonly used decongestants include pseudoephedrine and phenylephrine. These medications may be found alone or more frequently in combination with other medications under many brand names (see page 240). While phenylpropanolamine (PPA) was used in many popular sinus remedies, the FDA ordered all PPA products withdrawn because of a suspected link to stroke in young women.

There can be a downside to decongestants. As they stimulate the nervous system, they are known to cause light-headedness, increased heart rate and blood pressure, insomnia, and the jitters. To decrease the side effects of decongestants, try taking only the morning dose. Or cut the dose in half and see whether that gives relief without "speeding you up." If you use certain psychiatric medications such as Parnate, a monoamine oxidase (MAO) inhibitor used to treat severe depression, then talk with your doctor before taking any decongestant. Also get your doctor's consent before taking a decongestant if you have the following medical problems:

- Severe hypertension
- Coronary artery disease
- Hyperthyroidism
- Diabetes mellitus
- Prostate disease

Decongestants

ORAL

Generic Name	Brand Name
Pseudoephedrine	Sudafed, Novafed
Phenylephrine	

TOPICAL LONG-ACTING (8 TO 12 HOURS)

Generic Name	Brand Name
Oxymetazoline	Afrin
Xylometazoline	Neo-Synephrine 12-hour/maximum Sinex

TOPICAL SHORT-ACTING (3 TO 8 HOURS)

Generic Name	Brand Name
Tetrahydrozoline	
Naphazoline	Privine
Phenylephrine	Vicks, Duration, Neo-Synephrine

Antihistamines

Antihistamines are the first line of therapy for allergies, as they decrease itching, sneezing, and runny nose. Although they do *not* cure your allergy or end your congestion, they do block the effect of "histamine" and help relieve annoying symptoms. (Histamine is a substance in the body that causes nasal stuffiness and dripping in a cold or hay fever, bronchoconstriction in asthma, and itchy spots in a skin allergy; see page 29.) For sinus trouble, however, antihistamines may actually *worsen* the problem, causing the mucus to dry out and making it difficult to drain. Stagnant mucus can lead to an all-out sinus infection, so use caution with allergy medications that may slow cilia action.

If you have allergies, your doctor may prescribe short-acting antihistamines, taken every four to six hours, or timed-release antihistamines, taken every twelve hours. Based on scientific evidence, we know that these drugs work best if taken *before* allergy symptoms begin. In this regard the medications can build up in the blood if taken regularly for three to four days, giving a protective effect.

The most common side effects of antihistamines are sedation, drowsiness, and dry mouth. You may want to take any sedating antihistamine at night before bedtime to avoid feeling sluggish during the day. Some of the newer antihistamines—such as loratadine (Claritin), fexofenadine (Allegra), and cetirizine (Zyrtec)—are highly effective and unlikely to cause drowsiness or deleterious side effects.

Antihistamines have a *minimal* role in the treatment of sinusitis, as they can cause drying of mucous membranes and interfere with the clearing of secretions. Remember, you *want* to keep your mucus thin and moving! However, antihistamines are important for those who have allergy symptoms along with sinusitis.

Note: Before accepting *any* medication from your pharmacist, tell him or her about any other medication you are on, past reactions to medications, and your medical history—current or previous conditions, such as heart disease, high blood pressure, diabetes, or kidney disease. Carefully read and adhere to any in-

Antihistamines

NONSEDATING OR MILDLY SEDATING

Generic Name	Brand Name
Loratadine	Claritin
Cetirizine	Zyrtec
Fexofenadine	Allegra

SEDATING

Generic Name	Brand Name
Brompheniramine	Dimetane
Chlorpheniramine	Chlor-Trimeton
Diphenhydramine	Benadryl
Tripelennamine	PBZ
Promethazine	Phenergan
Azatadine	Optimine
Hydroxyzine	Atarax, Vistaril
Clemastine	Tavist
Cyproheptadine	Periactin

structions or warnings that appear on the label. If you have difficulty sleeping while taking allergy medicine, consider using Benadryl. This over-the-counter product helps to dry the nose and also causes drowsiness.

In Combination?

Many times a decongestant is not effective, and the combination of an antihistamine and a decongestant is more potent. In fact, many antihistamine-decongestant combinations are available today. Some products are targeted at stopping sinus swelling and congestion, along with pain relief. These products combine decongestants with pain relievers or combine antihistamines, decongestants, and expectorants with pain relievers. For example, Excedrin Sinus (tablet, caplet) combines the pain reliever acetaminophen with pseudoephedrine, a decongestant. Sinarest (tablet) adds the antihistamine chlorpheniramine to the combination of acetaminophen with pseudoephedrine (pain reliever plus decongestant). Both products work on different symptoms to bring you optimum relief. Be sure to check the ingredients, to see if they meet your personal needs, and the side effects, to make sure that the combination product is safe for you. Having one pharmacist who knows you and your medications is recommended and may help you to avoid toxic drug combinations.

ANTIBIOTIC USE OR OVERUSE?

Perhaps there is nothing more distressing than a patient who comes in and asks outright for an antibiotic even before the doctor has performed a physical examination or made a diagnosis. The problem is that antibiotics cure only certain bacteria-related illnesses—and if they are taken carelessly, you may get more serious health problems than you bargained for. With any illness, it is critical to address the underlying cause of the illness, whether it's bacterial or viral.

Astelin Nasal Spray Stops Postnasal Drip

Astelin nasal spray (azelastine) is indicated for the treatment of the symptoms of seasonal allergic rhinitis, such as rhinorrhea, sneezing, and nasal pruritus, in adults and children five years and older, and for treatment of the symptoms associated with vasomotor rhinitis, such as rhinorrhea, nasal congestion, and postnasal drip, in adults and children twelve years and older. Because Astelin is a histamine blocker, and steroid nasal sprays are more anti-inflammatory, some people do well by combining both sprays. Astelin should not be combined with oral antihistamines and may cause drowsiness.

Jenny was one patient who knew before she was even examined that an antibiotic would cure everything—even her chronic postnasal drip syndrome. This forty-year-old computer executive with a history of rhinosinusitis went to her doctor with symptoms of nasal congestion and purulent postnasal drip. She said these symptoms were "ruining her life," and she knew that the "right" antibiotic would resolve this within forty-eight hours. After all, her colleague had taken this antibiotic, and he was symptom-free within a few days.

Jenny's doctor told her that she would have to undergo a full examination and some lab tests before a diagnosis could be made—and even then, an antibiotic was probably not the answer to her problem.

Antibiotics can save people's lives, and if you need them,

you should get them as quickly as you can. Since only your doctor can prescribe antibiotics, this means that you should talk to your doctor if your think you might need antibiotics (as opposed to taking a family member's leftover pills from last winter's illness). However, it is the grave overreliance on and inappropriate use of these medications that have contributed to the global antibiotic resistance crisis that we face. Now it's time that we *all* become part of the solution.

A recent study by the U.S. Centers for Disease Control and Prevention found that many adults believe that if they are sick enough to see a doctor for a cold, they should get an antibiotic treatment. The study also found that patients are not aware of the consequences of taking the drugs if they are not needed. But when antibiotics are misused, bacteria can become resistant.

Some bacteria block the antibiotic's destructive capability by producing enzymes that render the drug ineffective. Other resistant bacteria may eliminate the drug's targets in bacterial cells, so the medications cannot work. When bacteria are repeatedly exposed to antibiotics, such as when you take the medication needlessly or too frequently, the germs in your body change. These changes can make the germs stronger than before, so they completely repel the antibiotic—and win. Your illness will linger with no signs of improvement. Or it may suddenly take a turn for the worse, requiring you to seek emergency medical care. You may have to be admitted to the hospital and get several different antibiotics administered intravenously. Sadly, those around you may get the resistant bacteria and come down with a similar illness that is very difficult to treat.

Consider that in 1954, 2 million pounds of antibiotics were produced in the United States. Today, that figure exceeds 50 million pounds. Many doctors claim to write prescriptions simply to meet patient demands; more than 50 million of the 150 million antibiotic prescriptions written each year for patients outside of hospitals are unnecessary, according to a CDC study. There is a way to protect yourself and others from resistant bacteria—and that is to respect antibiotics and take them only when necessary for a bacterial infection.

After examining Anne, her doctor found that she did *not* have an infection—but she did have nasal polyps, outgrowths of the mucosal lining of the nose that are common in patients with allergic rhinitis (congestion resulting from allergy), sinusitis, hay fever, and asthma. The polyps are benign, but they can cause chronic nasal congestion, difficulty breathing through the nose, and a perpetual runny nose with postnasal drip syndrome. Her doctor said that antibiotics would not resolve the trigger of her postnasal drip—nasal polyps. Instead, he prescribed a short burst (one week) of oral corticosteroids to reduce the size of the polyps. This treatment was followed by regular usage of a nasal steroid spray (pages 252–253). Her doctor also recommended that Anne use regular nasal saline irrigation, as discussed in Step 2, to help the mucus run freely so bacteria would not have a place to breed.

Though she was disappointed that she did not receive an antibiotic, Anne started the program to manage the nasal polyps. Within a week, she was feeling better—the congestion was resolved and she had less postnasal drip. One month later, Anne called to say her postnasal drip had stopped altogether.

Taking Antibiotics Responsibly

■ When you see your doctor, do not demand antibiotics. Your doctor will try to determine if you have a bacterial infection or a virus and will prescribe antibiotics only if necessary.

■ If your doctor prescribes antibiotics, don't be afraid to use them. While your body may develop resistant bacteria when you take antibiotics, after you finish your course of treatment, the nonresistant bacteria normally found in your system will return and compete with the resistant ones. As a result, the resistant bacteria may not exist in sufficient numbers to lead to illness.

■ Use antibiotics exactly as prescribed. Take the full course of treatment on time and as directed, and do not save pills "just in case" you might get sick later on. Safely discard any remaining pills in a way so that others, particularly children, cannot get access to them.

■ Do not give your antibiotics to anyone else, and do not take someone else's medication.

WHEN ANTIBIOTICS ARE NECESSARY TO KILL BACTERIA

An antibiotic is used if you have an increased amount of thick mucus or mucus that is colored (yellow, green, or brown). Yet because penetration of antibiotics into the sinuses is difficult due to poor blood supply, the medication may not get to the diseased tissue and bony material in your sinuses. Therefore, the required treatment is often a lengthy process—a minimum of two weeks and usually as long as six to eight weeks for some infections.

If you are not finding relief for a sinus infection within a few days, check back with your doctor to see whether the antibiotic is working for your particular infection. Certain bacteria have become resistant to some antibiotics in some locales, and stronger medications may be needed.

The specific antibiotic and the method of delivery are changing daily as doctors try to find the most effective and safest means to cure a sinus infection. Today, antibiotics can be taken orally, systemically (intravenously or by injection), or topically. In theory, they can also be delivered by a nebulizer. This portable machine is similar to the device hospitals use and turns liquid medication into a mist as it is inhaled into the lungs. A face mask or mouthpiece may be used depending on the patient's ability to inhale properly. The problem is that unless you've had sinus surgery and all sinuses are wide open, the medication does not end up in the sinus cavity. Antibiotics can also be delivered by a simple nasal spray. With this method, the medication appears to get to the infected area of the nose. Some doctors recommend that the prescribed antibiotics be added to the saline solution used with the Hydro Pulse Nasal/Sinus Irrigator (page 120). By removing thick phlegm that may block the antibiotic from reaching the sinus cavities, and by using the principles of suction and pumping action, the medication is quickly delivered into the sinuses, yet safely bypasses the lungs and other areas. An added safety factor is that a smaller amount of antibiotic needs to be used when compared to the dose taken orally.

Infections Caused by Viruses Do Not Need Antibiotics

- Colds
- Flu
- Most coughs and bronchitis
- Sore throats (except for strep throat)

Topical antibiotics such as Bactroban are also being used today. These topical ointments stay in contact with infected areas for long periods of time and clinically show a good effect on nasal infection. In some severe cases of chronic sinusitis, your doctor may have to use intravenous antibiotics to get to the root of the infection. IV antibiotics are delivered directly into the bloodstream, where they can reach the deepest infection and diseased tissues. This allows greater amounts of the medication to reach the infection.

Notify your doctor of any side effects experienced with any medication, such as a skin rash, increased breathing problems, or other symptoms. Antibiotics can also deplete your body of the necessary good bacteria. You can replace these by taking lactobacillus tablets, eating yogurt, or drinking sweet acidophilus milk.

Be sure to ask your doctor if reducing the bacteria load in your nose with nasal irrigation may help you reduce the duration of antibiotic treatment or even avoid it altogether.

Anticholinergics

Anticholinergics are particularly helpful for those with a clear, watery discharge (rhinorrhea) from the nose. These medications may work when antihistamines or other decongestants do not. The most effective one available today is ipratropium bromide (Atrovent), a topical spray that comes in two strengths. (The 0.03 percent preparation is useful for allergic and nonallergic rhinitis when the clear watery discharge is a prominent problem. Atrovent is also useful for vasomotor rhinitis [see pages 48–49]. The 0.06 percent strength is useful when a common cold caused by a virus produces postnasal drip.) The most common side effect is irritation or excessive nasal dryness, which can lead to nosebleeds.

Nasal Sprays

If you need immediate relief for a swollen, congested nasal passage, decongestant nasal sprays such as oxymetazoline (Afrin) and phenylephrine (Neo-Synephrine) can be helpful. Decongestant nasal sprays are safe to use to halt progression of sinus infections following colds or to prevent Eustachian tube problems when flying. Unlike oral decongestants (pills, liquids, capsules, tablets), *it is important to stop using decongestant nasal sprays after three to five days to avoid the development of rebound congestion or recurrent congestion.* Most of the sprays carry a warning, which should be read before usage.

Antibiotics Frequently Used for Sinus Infections

Generic Name	Brand Name
Amoxicillin	Amoxil
Amoxicillin and potassium clavulanate	Augmentin
Trimethoprim and sulfamethoxazole	Bactrim, Septra
Clarithromycin	Biaxin
Cefaclor	Ceclor
Ciprofloxacin	Cipro
Ofloxacin	Floxin
Telilthromycin	Ketek
Levofloxacin	Levaquin
Ampicillin	Omnipen
Penicillin and potassium	Pen Vee K
Tetracycline	Sumycin
Doxycycline	Vibramycin
Azithromycin	Zithromax

Steroids

Corticosteroids, which can be obtained by prescription only, are the most effective medications available for the treatment of sinus or nasal congestion as a result of allergy or nonallergic causes. With steroids the oral therapy (by mouth) is more effective and gets started more quickly than topical or inhaled usage. A seven- to ten-day course of prednisone is usually successful in controlling symptoms. Treatment with inhaled cromolyn or nasal steroids may follow this oral therapy.

Inhaled Steroids

At least six inhaled steroids are now available by prescription. Dexamethasone is the most potent, yet this drug may be absorbed in its active form and produce some serious side effects. The other drugs, however, are less likely to be absorbed and are metabolized or cleared quickly from the bloodstream if absorbed. They produce few, if any, side effects if taken in the recommended doses. Nasal irritation is the most common side effect. Sometimes this is severe enough to produce nasal bleeding. If this happens, stop taking the medicine immediately; perforation of the nasal septum can occur.

If you use an inhaled nasal steroid spray, do not spray the medication against your nasal septum. Instead, point the tip of the applicator toward the ear of the side you are spraying. Some of these drugs can be used once a day; the best time is about an hour before bedtime. If your nose has thick mucus, try irrigating first to get better drug contact with the nasal surface.

Many types of containers are available for inhaled sprays. Work with your doctor to find one that will work best for your condition. Usually these sprays can be taken for several months without a problem, but some doctors recommend that they be used for only five to fourteen days at a time. When your nasal congestion is relieved, you may stop the spray for a while before you need it again for another period of treatment.

Nasal Steroid Inhalers

Generic Name	Brand Name
Beclomethasone	Beconase, Vancenase
Budesonide	Rhinocort
Dexamethasone	Dexacort
Flunisolide	Nasalide, Nasarel
Fluticasone	Flonase
Mometasone	Nasonex
Triamcinolone	Nasacort

Leukotriene Inhibitors

Be sure to ask your doctor about leukotriene inhibitors (Accolate, Singulair), which are marketed for asthma and other lung diseases. These drugs work at the level of the cell receptors that ordinarily respond to leukotrienes, substances released from the membranes of mast cells during reactions mediated by immunoglobulin E (IgE) that cause uncomfortable bronchoconstriction and excessive secretion of mucus. The inhibitor medications keep the bronchial tubes from constricting. Allergies also cause leukotrienes to be active in other parts of the body, so these drugs may be effective in treating allergic conditions such as hives or sinusitis. Some researchers have found that this new type of medication may be almost as effective as steroids—without the side effects!

Drugs That Affect Mucus

A *mucokinetic agent* is a drug that helps thin the mucus to make it flow more easily. While many experts feel that water is most beneficial to help liquefy mucus, you can also use such medications as guaifenesin (Robitussin expectorant, Scot-Tussin expectorant, Humabid, Fenesin, Deconsal, Entex LA, Zephrex, and Dura-Vent). Sometimes guaifenesin must be used in high dosages, typically 2,400 milligrams per day. If you have asthma, make sure the expectorant does not contain antihistamine or cough suppressants unless prescribed by your doctor. The most common adverse effects of expectorants are nausea and vomiting.

Mast Cell Stabilizer

Cromolyn sodium (Nasalcrom) is a mast cell stabilizer that *prevents* allergic reactions in the nasal passage. This spray blocks the allergy response and is used even when you are symptom-free. Nasalcrom is available over the counter at most grocery stores and drugstores. This is best started six weeks before the pollen season. Ask your doctor if this would work in your situation.

WHAT ABOUT SINUS HEADACHE?

The experience of sinus pain—from the dull aching in your eyes to the misery of swollen glands to sharp pains in your ears from trapped fluid—is universal. If you suffer with sinus pain, you've probably lived on aspirin, acetaminophen, or traditional non-steroidal anti-inflammatory drugs (NSAIDs) to end the pain and allow you to live a halfway normal life.

Acetaminophen (Tylenol) is a pain reliever—but not in the same category as aspirin or traditional NSAIDs. It is the only pain reliever that will *not* cause stomach upset and gastrointestinal bleeding. Acetaminophen is a good treatment for mild to moderate pain, but it has the side effect of possibly causing liver damage, especially if taken with alcohol.

Besides aspirin, NSAIDs are the most heavily used drugs in the world. These medications work as anti-inflammatory agents and pain relievers. Today more than fifty NSAIDs are available. These "wonder drugs" give the benefits of high-dose aspirin with fewer side effects. With each one there is an individual response in pain control and possibility of side effects. Yet while these traditional NSAIDs can relieve pain and stiffness, they still leave the problems of stomach and kidney damage for many.

The Downside of NSAIDs

Aspirin sensitivity occurs in about 10 to 15 percent of people with asthma and 30 to 40 percent of those who have asthma and nasal polyps. While not truly an "allergy," aspirin sensitivity is a reaction similar to reactions to IV contrast dyes used in CT scans. Some of the symptoms you may feel include itching, rashes, hives, and swelling. Or you may have itchy/watery eyes, nasal congestion, cough, difficulty breathing, and wheezing. *Note:* Before you take aspirin or an NSAID, talk with your doctor to make sure this will not hurt you. Although NSAIDs relieve pain and swelling, there can be serious side effects. NSAIDs increase the risk for hospitalization and death from gastrointestinal bleeding or stomach or intestinal perforation from peptic ulcer.

If you are careful to watch for side effects, then sometimes

Analgesics Commonly Used to Relieve Pain

Analgesic—Generic Name	Product—Brand Name
Ibuprofen	Advil*
Naproxen	Aleve*
Aspirin and caffeine	Anacin*
Acetaminophen	Anacin-3
Acetaminophen	Anacin Maximum Strength
Buffered aspirin	Ascriptin*
Aspirin	Bayer*
Buffered aspirin	Bufferin*
Aspirin, acetaminophen, and caffeine	Excedrin Extra-Strength*
Ibuprofen	Motrin-IB*
Aspirin	Norwich*
Ibuprofen	Nuprin*
Ketoprofen	Orudis*
Acetaminophen	Tylenol
Aspirin, acetaminophen, and caffeine	Vanquish*

*Should be used with caution by those with nasal polyps.

NSAIDs can be taken over a long period of time. If your doctor wants you to stay on an NSAID, see whether a medication to prevent peptic ulcers would be helpful in your case. The following medications are taken differently, depending on the severity of your stomach problem. Your doctor can prescribe the most effective medication and treatment regime.

Common Side Effects of NSAIDs

- Abdominal pain
- Abnormal liver tests (blood tests)
- Asthma in those who are allergic to NSAIDs
- Diminishment of the effect of diuretics
- Dizziness
- Gastritis
- Heartburn
- Increased blood pressure (hypertension)
- Indigestion
- Intestinal bleeding
- Kidney (renal) failure or aggravation of renal failure
- Lower hemoglobin (anemia)
- Peptic ulcer
- Possibility of affecting other medications taken
- Possibility of decreasing platelet count (which can affect bleeding)
- Ringing in the ears (tinnitus)

IMMUNOTHERAPY FOR REDUCING ALLERGY AND ASTHMA SYMPTOMS

If you find that the medications you are taking are not effective in reducing allergy and asthma symptoms, your doctor may suggest allergy shots (injections or immunotherapy). Allergy shots are effective for reducing allergic symptoms associated with cat dander, pollens, house dust mites, certain molds, and fire ant

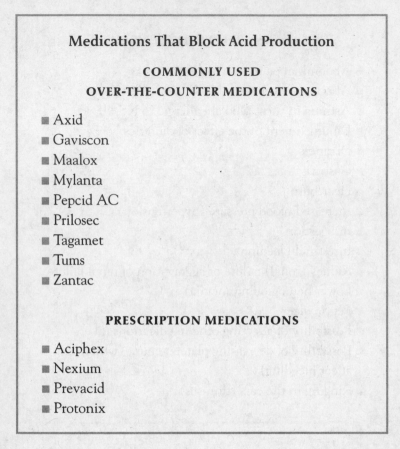

Medications That Block Acid Production

COMMONLY USED
OVER-THE-COUNTER MEDICATIONS

- Axid
- Gaviscon
- Maalox
- Mylanta
- Pepcid AC
- Prilosec
- Tagamet
- Tums
- Zantac

PRESCRIPTION MEDICATIONS

- Aciphex
- Nexium
- Prevacid
- Protonix

bites. Regular injections of allergens, given in increasing doses, stimulate changes in the immune system that decrease the chance of future allergic reactions.

Once your physician has helped you to identify the allergens that trigger symptoms through medical history and allergy testing, a series of injections with solutions containing increasing concentrations of these allergens may be used to lessen your sensitivity and reduce symptoms. These shots, which are the only known way to turn off allergic disease, reduce the production of IgE and cause the body to make another class of antibody called blocking-IgG. The blocking-IgG antibody actually helps protect you from allergic diseases. Shots are the only method available for long-lasting protection from allergies, particularly allergic rhinitis.

Studies have found that 85 percent of the people who receive allergy shots to treat hay fever due to grass, ragweed, trees, and dust get better. Your doctor will give shots of weak allergen solutions once or twice a week initially, then gradually increase the strength of the solution. When you reach the strongest dosage, you may receive the injections only once a month. The results are not immediate; estimates are that it takes three to five years to reach an optimal benefit. Many people get better for years, and some even permanently!

FINDING WHAT WORKS

Take advantage of the myriad new medical treatments. There are enough choices that most people should find something to help them breathe better. Talk about these options with your doctor and, together, decide on the most effective treatment combination that works best for your sinus condition and allows for greater activity and enjoyment of life.

Chapter 11

WHAT IF YOUR DOCTOR SAYS . . . SURGERY?

You've tried the alternative treatments, the prescribed medications . . . *still* you suffer with persistent, chronic sinusitis or infection. Don't worry; you are not alone. There are more options to consider, and while the final step—using surgical cures—is more invasive, it may help to finally resolve your sinus battle once and for all.

When sinusitis is chronic and will not clear up using various antibiotics and nasal drainage, your doctor may recommend surgery. Before you sign on the dotted line, you need to know that there is *no* such thing as minor surgery—even sinus surgery. There is always the chance of unexpected problems with any invasive procedure.

MAKING THE SURGERY DECISION

To decide if you are a good candidate for surgery, you must consider the specific sinus problems you have and how these have affected your quality of life. If your pain and congestion occur

What Types of Problems Can Surgery Correct?

WHEN SURGERY IS INDICATED

- When infection is due to diseased tissue and can't be cleared except by removal of the diseased tissue.
- When polyps block the sinuses and don't respond to medication.
- When there is a long history of sinus infection and the CT scan shows an anatomical blockage of the maxillary, ethmoid, and frontal sinuses.
- When you do not respond to medical management because the infected material can't get out of the sinus.
- When a bad tooth has caused major tissue changes.
- When repeated sinus infections are aggravating a chest condition—bronchitis, asthma, and others.

WHEN SURGERY IS NOT INDICATED

- If an MRI is taken for an unrelated problem and shows sinus disease, yet you do not have a clear history of sinus disease. Sometimes the MRI is too sensitive and may show serious sinus disease when in reality only mucus is present.
- When a sinus infection does not respond to antibiotics, yet the CT scan is not too bad. You may respond to office treatment to clear sinuses or try daily pulsatile nasal irrigation.

- When you can't breathe and a CT scan shows thickening of the membrane. If the physical examination shows that the nose looks allergic, you may respond to allergy management without surgery.
- When symptoms result from overuse of nose drops. These symptoms can be treated without surgery.

most of the time, and your quality of life is limited even with good medical treatment, then surgery may be a consideration. Or, if you have a serious anatomical problem that will not resolve without surgery, then this may be the only way to get well.

Before your doctor performs any surgery, a complete evaluation, including a detailed interview and physical examination (as discussed in chapter 4), will be done to see if you are a candidate.

SURGICAL CORRECTION— SOMETIMES THE ONLY CURE

In severe sinus disease, the regular anatomy may be distorted, and the only way to correct this is surgically. Nasal polyps may thin the bones, so a surgical procedure to remove the polyps can alleviate this problem. Or infectious swelling may move a structure in the sinus cavity to a different place, adding to your sinus misery.

If your doctor has mentioned surgery to you, yet you are still not convinced that this is a good idea, see the chart on page 261. This chart is a self-test that can help you determine whether sinus surgery is necessary. To use this hands-on method, chart the days on the calendar when your sinus problems keep you from living a normal life—from eating properly, sleeping, exercising, doing your daily tasks, and so on. During this time continue the treatments listed in chapters 5 to 10, including the medications and inhalers your doctor has prescribed.

After you have circled your bad sinus days, evaluate the calendar at the end of two months. If more days are circled than not, or if the sinus problems have not been resolved or have even worsened over this time, this may be an indication that surgery is warranted.

Whom to Call

To guarantee surgical success, a critical evaluation of the upper airway by a board-certified ear, nose, and throat surgeon (ENT or otolaryngologist) is the first step. Your ear, nose, and throat specialist has trained four to five years in this field after medical school and understands how anatomical problems can prevent your sinuses from being healthy.

The ENT doctor will take a thorough history of your symptoms and medical problems, then do a careful physical examination (see chapter 4). The doctor will use a fiber-optic scope to visualize the interior of the nose and a CT scan to image the sinus cavities and related anatomy.

Once your surgeon has determined the possible sites causing obstruction or problems, then the specific type of surgery will be explained. Surgery is performed only *after* the risks and benefits are fully discussed and the complementary and medical options described in chapters 5 to 10 have been exhausted without success. Because the surgical procedures have imposing names, and the anatomy of your upper airway is extremely intricate, it is

Sinus Calendar: Month 1

1	2	3	4	5	6	7
8	9	10	11	12	13	14
15	16	17	18	19	20	21
22	23	24	25	26	27	28
29	30	31				

Sinus Calendar: Month 2

1	2	3	4	5	6	7
8	9	10	11	12	13	14
15	16	17	18	19	20	21
22	23	24	25	26	27	28
29	30	31				

important that you ask many questions in order to understand how the operation(s) may help, as well as the possible risk factors.

SINONASAL ENDOSCOPY

Sinonasal endoscopy is a commonly used method for diagnosing and treating sinusitis. This painless procedure is done without anesthesia and involves guiding a tiny scope up into the nasal passages and sinuses to allow the doctor to see any obstructions, blockages, or infections. If infection is detected, the doctor can take a sample of the pus and culture this in the laboratory so the most effective treatment can be prescribed.

To complete a sinus examination, a CT scan of the sinuses is needed to show areas of the sinus anatomy not visualized by endoscopy. The scan can show specific blockages of the openings of the frontal, maxillary, ethmoid, and sphenoid sinuses. Using visualization by endoscope, the doctor can perform minimally invasive surgery using various instruments if blockages are found. Since no outer bone has been removed, there are no incisions in the face and much less trauma to the patient.

BALLOON SINUPLASTY

The basic principle of sinus therapy is to open the sinuses to allow drainage. Even severely diseased sinuses clear when drainage is established. With balloon sinuplasty, a groundbreaking new procedure that works for the sinuses as angioplasty does for the heart, doctors use endoscopy to guide a flexible balloon catheter through the nostrils into the sinus opening. Once in place, the balloon is gently inflated to restructure and widen the walls of the blocked passageway, allowing the sinuses to function normally.

So far, the results are quite promising, and the risks involved are minimal compared to other more invasive types of surgery.

The Most Common Sinus Problems That Require Surgery

Some common nasal conditions that can add to the severity of your chronic sinusitis include nasal valve collapse, septal deviation, enlarged turbinates, and nasal polyps. Nasal tumors are not common, but they, too, can be a cause of chronic sinus problems. Specific surgical procedures exist to correct each of these problems, and understanding how they work is important. Your doctor will decide which procedure is best for your situation.

DEVIATED SEPTUM

A *deviated septum* is one cause of sinusitis. It occurs when the cartilage and bone of your nasal septum have bent into the airway, causing obstruction and increased resistance to airflow. This condition may be hereditary or caused by trauma. A severe deviation of the septum may cause your nose to be stopped up day and night, resulting in snoring or disturbed sleep.

Surgery to correct the deviation, called *septoplasty*, structurally opens and widens the nasal airway and is performed in an operating room under general anesthesia or local anesthesia with sedation. The operation is usually done on an outpatient basis and lasts about 1½ hours.

The surgeon almost always performs septoplasty through the nose, without an external incision. If you are also having rhinoplasty done at the same time, there will be an incision. If your septum is severely deviated, the surgeon may remove portions of it, readjust the septum, and then reinsert the pieces into the nose.

Because the surgery is done inside your nose by removing or straightening the bent cartilage, there is no change to the external appearance of your nose, and you will have no visible bruising or swelling. You may go home the same day and experience very little pain or discomfort. If there is any bleeding, your nose may be packed for a day or two until this is controlled.

If your external nose is crooked, you will require *rhinoplasty* to straighten it. This can be done in conjunction with septoplasty. In septoplasty your surgeon will straighten the septum that is obstructing your airway or drainage and reset this into the midline of your nose. If your external nose needs to be cosmetically altered, it's a good idea to get both procedures done at the same time. Talk with your surgeon about your situation.

NASAL VALVE COLLAPSE

Nasal valve collapse refers to the collapse of the cartilage supporting the tip of the nose. When you breathe in and the cartilage is too weak to hold up against the airflow, the airway collapses. This is seen frequently in older people and in those who have had cosmetic surgery on the nose (rhinoplasty).

If you have nasal valve collapse, your doctor may recommend *nasal reconstruction*. This involves surgically adding cartilage to the nasal tip and is performed in an operating room under general or local anesthesia. Cartilage is taken from your nasal septum or your ear and used to support the nasal tip. This prevents further collapse and improves the nasal airway.

TURBINATE HYPERTROPHY

Enlargement of the turbinates, the spongy tissue inside your nose that swells and secretes mucus, can also cause nasal obstruction, leading to chronic, persistent sinusitis. Whether turbinate enlargement is caused by allergy, irritation, or chronic infection, it makes it difficult to breathe. Continued irritation of the turbinates, known as *rhinitis*, causes prolonged enlargement (*turbinate hypertrophy*) and leads to nasal obstruction.

Turbinate hypertrophy is treated in various ways. Yet care is needed to ensure that minimal damage is done to the skin covering the turbinate. Simply cutting off the turbinate will remove the beneficial function of the mucosa to warm and moisten the air before it gets to the lungs and to protect against infection.

Some approaches to treating turbinate hypertrophy are:

- *Submucus resection*. Here only the bone under the turbinate is disturbed, allowing the turbinate to be moved to the side, to improve the airway. This reduces the size as well.
- *Partial turbinectomy*. This involves the removal of parts of the turbinate that are diseased or nonfunctional.
- *Somnoplasty*. Here radio-frequency waves are used to reduce the vascular channel under the skin without disturbing the functions of the turbinate. This may require more than one office procedure.

NASAL POLYPS

Nasal polyps are grapelike swellings of the nasal tissue associated with allergy and irritation. In most cases polyps are benign (noncancerous) tissue but should be removed because they cause nasal obstruction and block your sinuses, predisposing them to infection.

Empty Nose Syndrome (ENS)

The turbinates, or shelves on the side of the nose, warm and moisten the air as it passes to the lungs. These turbinates have a large surface area so that the air you breathe in can pick up moisture and warmth. If these turbinates are removed in order to make more room for breathing or have been damaged so they no longer occupy previous space, then the nose "looks empty." In this condition the patient constantly feels like he or she is not getting enough air. The nose is dry, the air entering the lungs is cold, and the patient is quite miserable. Because there is no good long-term treatment, many patients get severely depressed.

To prevent empty nose syndrome, be sure your doctor does not perform surgery that reduces the function of your nasal cilia. Be wary of those professionals who promote "laser cures" for whatever nasal problem you have. If your doctor doesn't know what empty nose syndrome is, find an experienced doctor who does.

Without cilial function, use of nasal irrigation and moisturizing gels help breathing. With empty nose syndrome, you might be sensitive to benzalkonium preservatives and should consider using saline sprays with electrolytes that are preservative-free. Patients with ENS should carry a spray bottle of enhanced saline to use after odor or dust exposure.

Polyps are removed in an operating room under general anesthesia or local anesthesia with sedation. The procedure is done through your nose using the same technique as for correcting a deviated septum (see pages 266–67). Remember, polyps usually return even *after* surgery. So make sure you have tried all medical treatments before undergoing surgery for polyp removal.

NASAL TUMORS

Nasal tumors rarely occur, but when they do, they may cause nasal obstruction. Tumors may be benign (noncancerous) or malignant (cancerous) and are diagnosed by a complete nasal examination. Surgical removal of the tumor eliminates the obstruction and cures your snoring.

TONSILLECTOMY AND ADENOIDECTOMY

The tonsils and adenoids are made of lymphoid tissue and are part of the immune system. The tonsils are located on the side of the throat, while the adenoids are located behind the nose and above the soft palate. The tonsils and adenoids act as filters guarding the entrance to the lower respiratory system. They remove viruses, bacteria, and particles in the air. Sometimes they become clogged, swollen, and infected. In the 1960s, adenoid and tonsil enlargement was recognized as a cause of sleep apnea and snoring. Since that time, many reports have documented very large tonsils and adenoids as the cause of airway obstruction and snoring in adults and children.

Adenoid enlargement resulting in nasal obstruction is the most common cause of ear blockage and ear infections, as well as snoring in children. Extreme enlargement of the tonsils can cause snoring and sleep apnea, and is the most common cause of sleep apnea in children. The tonsils, adenoids, or both are removed if they are chronically infected or contribute to sleep apnea. Removal usually stops the snoring and decreases the apnea. However, the tonsils and adenoids are usually not removed for snoring alone.

Doctors can perform tonsillectomy and adenoidectomy in the operating room under general anesthesia. Both the tonsils and adenoids are removed through the mouth. The tonsils are removed by cutting the tissue away from the underlying muscle, using an electric cautery, laser, snare, or knife. All methods give similar results. Adenoids are removed by a specially designed instrument that passes through the mouth into the nose. Both procedures carry the risk of bleeding.

SURGICAL COMPLICATIONS

No matter what anyone tells you, no surgery is "minor." Even surgical procedures performed in an outpatient facility without general anesthesia carry some degree of risk. That's why it's important to make sure you have tried every treatment available before you agree to an invasive procedure. You should also consider the following complications before you agree to surgery:

■ *Dry mucous membranes.* A distressing complication of sinus surgery is that the mucous membranes may be dry for some time after the procedure. Because of the excessive removal of tissue, there are fewer mucus-making cells to produce the normal amount of mucus the body needs to stay healthy.

- *The nose being open too wide.* Another problem occurs if too much bone and cartilage are removed, leaving the nose open too much. When this happens, patients complain of burning and a dry feeling. This is very difficult to correct and a real problem with some surgeries.

- *Damage to blood vessels or muscles near the eyes.* Because the sinuses are next to the eyes, there may be excessive thinning of the bone or other changes that can cause the surgeon to enter your eye socket. Fortunately, there is still a bit of space before you reach the eye itself, but sometimes vessels or muscles can be damaged and blindness can occur.

- *Loss of sense of smell or leak of cerebrospinal fluid.* At the roof of the nose is an area where the skull dips down. Sometimes the dip is minimal; sometimes it is severe. If you've had chronic infections, there may be less bone that separates the nose and upper sinuses from the brain and brain contents. If a surgical opening is made into the skull, you may experience a loss of smell and a leak of fluid from the skull (called cerebrospinal fluid). If this problem is diagnosed right away, it can be fixed. However, if it is neglected, the leakage can result in infection in the brain area, including meningitis.

- *Missing diseased tissue.* Probably one of the most distressing complications comes when insufficient surgery is done. Somehow an area of diseased tissue is missed by the surgeon, and sinus symptoms persist, often requiring further surgery.

- *Bleeding after surgery.* Postoperative bleeding can occur, but this can be controlled, often in the doctor's office. There may be pain after surgery, but this is regularly controlled by medication.

■ *Nerve damage*. Most surgery today is done with telescopes through the nose. Sometimes it is necessary to do a Caldwell-Luc-type procedure. This procedure is performed by incising the gums and going into the maxillary sinus from the front of the cheek. Complications arise when the nerve of sensation to this cheek area is injured, leaving that area numb.

The Low Incidence of Complications

The good news is that most of these complications are rare. To further reduce the incidence of any such complications, a new procedure called Insta Trak was pioneered at Cedars Sinai Hospital by Martin Hopp, M.D. With Insta Trak a CT scan is taken with markers. Then, during surgery, the position of the instrument is displayed on an enlarged screen in three positions. The surgeon will see in these three views the instrument in relation to the important anatomical areas like the eye and the brain, resulting in fewer complications.

PREPARING FOR SURGERY

If you and your doctor decide that the final option for curing sinusitis is surgery, then it's important to know that each type of surgery described earlier has a specific advantage, depending on the severity and location of the problem and such factors as your age or other chronic illnesses. No matter how "minor" the procedure appears, you will still be expected to follow the doctor's orders as you recover. Plus, even after the surgery, you will still need to take measures to keep your sinuses healthy—using nasal irrigation, if recommended, getting healing sleep, eating healthful nutrients, and taking prescribed medications or using inhalers.

Make sure your CT films will be available in the operating room when the surgeon does the procedure. These films show any unusual anatomy and help to guide the surgeon correctly. If you are coming down with the flu or have an infection, consider delaying the surgery, and be sure you have stopped taking blood-thinning products or herbs that can cause blood thinning (see pages 148, 151–152) far enough in advance.

Finally, let your doctor guide you as you choose which type of surgery is best to help you end sinus pain and discomfort and regain an active life. Good luck!

NOTES

Chapter 1 What Is Sinusitis?

1. Yonkers AJ. Sinusitis—inspecting the causes and treatment. *Ear Nose Throat J*. 1992;71:258.
2. Snow V et al. Position paper endorsed by the American Academy of Family Physicians, the American College of Physicians—American Society of Internal Medicine, and the Infectious Diseases Society of America. *Ann Intern Med*. 2001; 134:495.
3. *NIH Data Book 1990*. Bethesda, MD: US Department of Health and Human Services, 1990. Pub. #90-1261. Table 44.
4. Gliklich RE, Metson R. The health impact of chronic sinusitis in patients seeking otolaryngologic care. *Otolaryngol Head Neck Surg*. 1995;113:104.
5. Kirkpatrick GL. The common cold. *Prim Care*. 1996;23:657.
6. Berg O, Carenfelt C, Rystedt G, Änggård A. Occurrence of asymptomatic sinusitis in common cold and other acute ENT infections. *Rhinology* 1986;24:223.
7. Allergies in America: A Landmark Survey of Nasal Allergy

Sufferers. Available at: www.myallergiesinamerica.com. Accessed March 20, 2006.

Chapter 2   Sinusitis and Coexisting Problems

1. National Asthma Education Program Expert Panel. Guidelines for the diagnosis and management of asthma. National Institutes of Health, Bethesda, MD, 1991, Pub. #91-3042.

Chapter 5   Step 2: Try Nasal Irrigation

1. Subiza JL, Subiza J, Barjau MC, Rodríguez R, Gavilán MJ. Inhibition of the seasonal IgE increase to *Dactylis glomerata* by daily sodium chloride nasal-sinus irrigation during the grass pollen season. *J Allergy Clin Immunol.* 1999;104(3):711–12.

Chapter 6   Step 3: Consider Complementary Treatments

1. Akhondzadeh S, Kashani L, Mobaseri M, Hosseini SH, Nikzad S, Khani M. Passionflower in the treatment of opiates withdrawal: a double-blind randomized controlled trial. *Journal of Clinical Pharmacy and Therapeutics.* 2001 Oct;26(5):369–73.

Chapter 8   Step 5: Boost Healing Nutrients

1. Macheix J, Fleuriet A, Billot J. *Fruit Phenolics.* Boca Raton, FL: CRC Press, 1990.
2. Lazze MC, Pizzala R, Savio M, et al. Anthocyanins protect against DNA damage induced by tert-butyl-hydroperoxide in rat smooth muscle and hepatoma cells. *Mutat Res.* 2003; 535(1):103–15.
3. Roy S, Khanna S, Alessio HM, et al. Anti-angiogenic property of edible berries. *Free Radic Res.* 2002;36(9):1023–31.

GLOSSARY

Acupuncture: Ancient stress reliever that uses needles to puncture the skin at certain points on the body. Acupuncture helps to stimulate the body's natural defenses and alter the activity of the immune system.

Allergens: Substances such as dust that trigger the body's allergic reaction and cause the nose to run or become congested.

Allergy: An overreaction of the immune system to an ordinarily harmless substance known as an allergen.

Antibiotics: Drugs that kill bacteria or slow down their reproduction. By doing this, they help the body's own immune defenses such as the white blood cells and various antibodies to clear bacteria from the body.

Antibodies: Specific types of proteins, called immunoglobulins, which are part of the body's defense mechanism. Antibodies are made to neutralize a foreign protein in the body.

Apnea: The cessation of breathing that may occur during sleep.

Asthma: Refers to a disease marked by sudden, repeated attacks of shortness of breath due to narrowing of the bronchi. There may also be wheezing and cough.

Bronchi: The airways that connect the windpipe (trachea) to the lungs.

Bronchioles: The smaller airways in the lungs.

Bronchoconstriction: A narrowing of the bronchial airways that may cause wheezing or difficulty breathing.

Bronchodilator: A drug that widens and relaxes the bronchi.

Chiropractic: Manipulation of the spine in order to alleviate symptoms and promote healing of all sorts of medical disorders as well as muscular and bone injuries; may help relieve sinus headache.

CPAP: A commonly used abbreviation for *continuous positive airway pressure*, which is used to relieve the obstruction in the oropharynx in patients with OSA.

CT scan: A commonly used abbreviation for computed tomography, which is a special type of X-ray imaging technique for getting detailed information about the anatomy in a particular part of the body such as the sinuses.

Detoxification: The act of cleansing the body of toxins—purification of the human body, mind, and spirit.

Dyspnea: Shortness of breath, a feeling of breathlessness, or a sense of not getting enough air that is out of proportion to activity.

Endoscope: A highly flexible instrument used to make an accurate diagnosis.

Eosinophils: A type of white blood cell associated with allergic diseases.

Essential fatty acids (EFAs): Not manufactured by the body, but are essential to health and normal brain development.

Found in fish oils and in plant oils such as evening primrose, black currant, and borage.

Herb: A plant or part of a plant that can be used in medicine or seasoning.

Histamine: A substance in the body that causes nasal stuffiness and dripping during a cold or hay fever, bronchoconstriction in asthma, and itchy spots in a skin allergy.

Homeopathy: Naturopathic form of medicine that helps reduce allergic rhinitis, hay fever, migraine headaches, trauma, gastritis, allergic asthma, acute childhood diarrhea, fibromyalgia, and influenza.

Hydrotherapy: Any rehabilitative therapy that involves soaking in water, usually warm whirlpool baths.

Hypothyroidism: A condition in which the thyroid, a gland located under the skin in front of your neck, secretes abnormally low amounts of active hormone into the blood. This causes the body to use energy from food more slowly than normal, causing problems of weight gain or difficulty in losing weight.

Immune system: Cells and proteins that work to protect the body from harmful, infectious microorganisms such as bacteria, viruses, and fungi.

Immunoglobulin E (IgE):   The most important antibody during an allergic reaction. Everyone makes IgE; however, people who have a genetic predisposition toward allergy make larger quantities of this protective protein.

Immunotherapy: A form of allergy treatment to prevent reactions to pollens, dust mites, mold, insects, and animal dander. The person is given gradually increasing doses of the allergen or substance to which he or she is allergic, making the immune system less sensitive or reactive.

Insomnia: A condition in which the person complains of difficulty falling asleep or problems staying asleep.

Larynx: The organ of voice production, located in the upper part of the respiratory system between the pharynx and the trachea. It includes the vocal cords.

Laser: A device that produces a beam of high-energy light that can be used to shrink or burn tissue during a surgical procedure such as the reduction in size of the uvula and soft palate.

Lungs: The main part of the respiratory system that takes oxygen from the air into the bloodstream and allows carbon dioxide to escape from the body.

Mast cells: Allergy-causing cells in the mucous lining of the nose, sinuses, and bronchi. They contain chemicals such as histamine.

MRI: A commonly used abbreviation for *magnetic resonance imaging*. MRI does not involve the use of radiation as in X-rays but may be very useful in looking at a particular structure in the body.

Mucokinetic agent: A drug that helps thin mucus to make it easier to flow.

Mucous membrane: A soft, pink, skin-like structure that lines many cavities and tubes in the body, such as the respiratory tract. The mucous membrane secretes a fluid containing mucus.

Mucus: A viscid, slippery secretion produced by the mucous membrane, which helps to lubricate and protect certain parts of the body.

Olfaction: The word for smell.

OSA: A commonly used abbreviation for *obstructive sleep apnea*.

Placebo effect: A reaction that refers to the mysterious and uncharted mechanisms by which the power of suggestion can result in a physiological change; usually refers to case studies where participants are given "sugar pills" rather than the actual studied product.

Pulmonary: Relating to the lungs.

Rhinitis: The technical term used for a running or congested nose. *Rhino-* refers to the nose and *-itis* means inflammation or swelling.

Rhonchi: Whistling or snoring sounds heard through the stethoscope when listening to the chest. Rhonchi indicate partial obstruction of the airways by mucus or other inflammatory debris such as pus.

Snoring: The noise produced by vibration of the soft palate and uvula.

Supplement: Substances to be added to a diet weak in essential nutrients, vitamins, and minerals. Available in different forms such as capsules, caplets, and pills.

Tonsils: Structures located on both sides of the oropharynx that may cause narrowing of the airway if enlarged.

Tonsoliths: White exudate on the tonsils.

Triggers: The factors that cause an allergy, sinus, or asthma attack by initiating airway inflammation.

Turbinates: Tubular structures that project into the nasal chambers and increase the surface area of the walls inside the nose. A mucous membrane that is rich in blood vessels covers these turbinates. The turbinates may swell and cause nasal obstruction.

Uvula: A cone-shaped projection hanging down from the soft palate in the oropharynx. The uvula may become swollen and enlarged in people who snore.

Vaccine: A preparation given to induce immunity against an infectious disease. Most vaccines contain weakened versions of the specific organisms against which immunity is sought. They do not cause the disease but stimulate the body's immune response to the infectious agent.

Wheeze: The sound heard during breathing that indicates an obstruction in the airways. It is usually heard during expiration but can be heard sometimes during inspiration.

REFERENCES

Allergies in America: A Landmark Survey of Nasal Allergy Sufferers. Available at: www.myallergiesinamerica.com. Accessed Mar 20, 2006.

American Dietetic Association 1997 Nutrition Trends Survey. American Dietetic Association, September 1997.

Bartels CL, Miller SJ. Herbal and related remedies. *Nutrition in Clinical Practice*. 1998;12(2):5–19.

Berg O, Carenfelt C, Rystedt G, Änggård A. Occurrence of asymptomatic sinusitis in common cold and other acute ENT-infections. *Rhinology*. 1986;24:223.

Borysenko J. *Minding the Body, Mending the Mind*. Reading, MA: Addison-Wesley, 1987, 10.

Callahan M. Antioxidants and fewer health problems. *Bottom Line Personal*. Jan 15, 1996, 8.

Chandra RK. Nutrition and the immune system: an introduction. *Am J Clin Nutr*. 1997;66(2):460S-463S.

Cohen S, Tyrrell DA, Smith AP. Psychological stress and susceptibility to the common cold. *N Engl J Med*. 1991;325: 606–12.

Conner BL et al. Magnetic resonance imaging of the paranasal sinuses: frequency and type of abnormalities. *Ann Allergy*. 1989 May;62(5):457–60.

Georgitis JW. Nasal hyperthermia and simple saline irrigation for perennial rhinitis, changes in inflammatory mediators. *Chest*. 1994;106:1487–82.

Gliklich RE, Metson R. The health impact of chronic sinusitis in patients seeking otolaryngologic care. *Otolaryngol Head Neck Surg*. 1995;113:104.

Grossan M. Asthma and sinusitis. www.emedicine.com/ent/topic516.htm.

———. Get natural relief from sinus misery. *Bottom Line Health*. Mar 5, 2002.

———. End ear pain. *Scuba Diving*. Jan 2004, 93–96.

———. Role of the mucociliary flow system in the treatment of sinus infection. *Today's Therapeutic Trends*. 2001; 19(3):205–12.

———. The ins and outs of common ear problems. *Patient Care*. Apr 2002, 56–71.

Kirkpatrick GL. The common cold. *Prim Care*. 1996;23:657.

McGrady A, Conran P, Dickey D, Garman D, Farris E. The effects of biofeedback-assisted relaxation on cell-mediated immunity, cortisol, and white blood cell count in healthy adult subjects. *Journal of Behavioral Medicine*. 1992;15(4): 343–54.

Merkus P. Classification of cilio-inhibiting effects of nasal drugs. *Laryngoscope*. 2001;111:595–601.

National Asthma Education Program Expert Panel. Guidelines for the diagnosis and management of asthma. Pub. #91-3042. National Institutes of Health, Bethesda, MD, 1991.

NIH Data Book 1990. Pub. #90-1261. Bethesda, MD: U.S. Department of Health and Human Services, 1990. Table 44.

Ozagar A et al. Aspiration of nasal secretions into the lungs in patients with acute sinonasal infections. *Laryngoscope.* 2000 Jan;110(1):107–10.

Parnes SM et al. Acute effects of antileukotrienes on sinonasal polyposis and sinusitis. *Ear Nose Throat J.* 2000 Jan;79(1): 18–20, 24–125.

Rachelevsky GS, Slavin RG et al. Sinusitis: acute, chronic and manageable. *Patient Care.* 1997;131:4.

Ramadan HH et al. Chronic rhinosinusitis and biofilms. *Otolaryngol Head Neck Surg.* 2005 Mar;132(3):414–17.

Reilly D et al. Is evidence for homeopathy reproducible? *Lancet.* 1994;344(8937):1601–6.

Scadding G. The effect of medical treatment of sinusitis upon concomitant asthma. *Allergy.* 1999;54 Suppl. 57:136–40.

Smolley L, Bruce D. *The Snoring Cure.* New York: Norton, 1999.
————. *Breathe Right Now.* New York: Dell, 1999.

Snow V et al. Position paper endorsed by the American Academy of Family Physicians, the American College of Physicians, American Society of Internal Medicine, and the Infectious Diseases Society of America. *Ann Intern Med.* 2001;134:495.

Spector SL, Nicklas RA. Practice parameters for the diagnosis and treatment of asthma. *J Allergy Clin Immunol* (Supplement). St. Louis: Mosby–Year Book, Inc., 1995.

Sridhar, MK. Nutrition and lung health: Should people at risk of obstructive lung disease eat more fruit and vegetables? *Br Med J.* 1995;310(6972):75–76.

Stenson, Jacqueline. Tai chi improves lung function in older people. Medical Tribune News Service. November 27, 1995.

Subiza JL et al. Sinus irrigation during the grass pollen season. *J Allergy Clin Immunol*. 1999;104(3 Pt 1):711–12.

Tomooka LT. Clinical study and literature review of nasal irrigation. *Laryngoscope*. 2000 Jul;110(7):1189–93.

Yonkers AJ. Sinusitis—inspecting the causes and treatment. *Ear Nose Throat J*. 1992;71:258.

INTERNET SITES THAT PROVIDE INFORMATION ON SINUSITIS

www.drdavidson.ucsd.edu. Informative Web site on sinusitis and other health problems provided by Dr. Terence Davidson of the Nasal Dysfunction Clinic, University of California at San Diego.

www.hydromedonline.com/presentingthehydropulse. Shows the Hydro Pulse method of pulsatile nasal irrigation.

http://healthlink.mcw.edu. Useful medical articles on sinusitis and related problems from the University of Wisconsin.

www.geocities.com/shouser144. Informative Web site with information on ear, nose, and throat problems.

www.ent-consult.com. Dr. Murray Grossan's Web site with information on all aspects of ear, nose, and throat and scuba medicine.

www.aaaai.org. Official Web site of the American Academy of Allergy, Asthma and Immunology.

www.sinuses.com. Informative Web site by Wellington S. Tichenor, M.D., a highly respected board-certified allergist.

www.aafa.org. Asthma and Allergy Foundation of America Web site with educational support groups.

www.aanma.org. Allergy and Asthma Network/Mothers of Asthmatics, Inc., Web site. This nonprofit organization provides support to parents of asthmatics.

www.entnet.org. American Academy of Otolaryngology—Head and Neck Surgery Web site with excellent information on all aspects of upper respiratory problems, including sinusitis.

www.aarc.org. American Association for Respiratory Care professionals Web site with educational resources for lay readers.

www.lungusa.org. American Lung Association Web site with educational material on lung problems and asthma.

www.nhlbi.nih.gov. National Heart Lung and Blood Institute Web site with the latest research on asthma, lungs, and the heart.

www.njc.org. National Jewish Medical and Research Center Hospital Web site devoted to allergy and asthma and related conditions.

www.earaid.info. This site discusses the use of antioxidants and nutrients.

Sources for Allergy Control Products
www.alerg.com
www.onlineallergyrelief.com/sinus/sinus.html
www.allergybuyersclub.com
www.natlallergy.com
www.allergycontrol.com
www.achooallergy.com
www.justnaturalstuff.co.uk
www.inmunotek.com

Sources for Breath Control Products
www.breathcure.com
www.dentist.net
www.just4teeth.com

INDEX

About the Authors

DEBRA FULGHUM BRUCE, PH.D., is an Atlanta-based health communications professional and former editor in chief of *Living Well Today*, a regional health and lifestyle publication. Dr. Bruce has written seventy-eight books, mostly health collaborations, with such major publishers as Ballantine, Bantam, Time Warner, Dell, Berkley, Macmillan USA, Simon & Schuster, Avon, Norton, Wiley, Dutton, ReganBooks, and more.

Among her latest books are *Making a Baby, Pain-Free Back, Pain-Free Arthritis*, and *The Fibromyalgia Handbook*.

Since 1970, MURRAY GROSSAN, M.D., a board-certified otolaryngologist and medical editor for this book, has specialized in treating patients who can't take ordinary drugs or have failed standard treatment. His successful non-drug method of using pulsatile nasal irrigation is detailed in *The Sinus Cure*. Dr. Grossan's Hydro Pulse Nasal/Sinus Irrigator was also featured in *Time* magazine's "Best Inventions." Dr. Grossan practices at Cedars-Sinai Medical Center in Los Angeles. His list of publications can be obtained at www.ent-consult.com/cv.html.